AN OUNCE OF PREVENTION

TESTIMONIES AND PRAISES FOR

"AN OUNCE OF PREVENTION"

Thank God for Drs. Atkins—
On August 21, 2008, I was diagnosed with Sjogren's disease. I also had fibrocystic breasts, headaches, thyroid disease, recurring Koeppe nodules in my left eye and restless nights. My wholistic counselor highly recommended Dr Pamela Atkins who put me on a healthy diet, herbal supplements and plenty of water. Dr Floyd coached me through their 40-Day Detox program in which I achieved much success. In just 3 months the results were 'FANTASTIC'! Most of my physical symptoms have gone away and I feel 100% better. If you are sick and in need of healing try this program. If you are healthy and want to maintain, then the Center for Wellness and Healing is the path that you must take.

Mildred Burnside
Houston, Texas

Hurricane Katrina brought me to the Wellness Center. I arrived with a diagnosis of prostate cancer by my urologist in New Orleans. I consulted with Doctors Atkins who suggested a change in diet, eating natural food, and replenishment of body with nutrients and supplements. Four years later, after careful and thoughtful recommendations, that I follow, I no longer experience symptoms of prostate problems. I also brought with me a diagnosis of congestive heart failure, and atrial fibrillation. And, as a heart patient the care from the doctors at the Wellness Center has prolonged my life for four years and I feel that my life following their suggested program will go on for another 10 or 15 years.

Silas H. Connor, 82-vibrant years old
Retired Teacher, School Administrator & General Contractor.
New Orleans, Louisiana

Dr. Floyd Atkins came to me with a new approach on life at a time when I desperately needed it. My high cholesterol was high and my blood sugar was out of control. I did not want to take any prescription drugs because of what I have seen my mother go through with a regiment of 12 different prescription drugs daily to maintain her health.

Dr. Atkins showed me how changes in my diet and my thinking could alleviate my problems. By following his recommendations, within months, my lab values were within normal range. Dr. Atkins has given me a whole new prospective on healthcare, medicine and just what prevention and wellness is all about. He can really make you see life clearly!

Walter Triche
Atlanta, Georgia

In June of 2008 I participated in Dr. Floyd's Six-Week Detox and Cleanse. This process involved eating a diet of fresh, organic fruits and vegetables, Wild Caught fish, while removing all partially hydrogenated oils, processed foods, refined sugars and dairy as well as other toxic chemicals. Aside from the aesthetic change, **I could not believe the mental clarity and the high energy level I was experiencing and without caffeine or candy**. After successful completion of the cleanse, I had a very clear understanding of the importance of the lifestyle change that would be necessary to maintain my weight loss and overall optimal health.

Sha'tu A'tyre Dailey
Fort Worth, Texas

"After completing the detox/cleansing and altering my eating habits, I was excited that my test results revealed that **my cholesterol decreased by 53 points** without any medication."

Greta Walter Fruge
Houston, Texas

"I had poor eating habits, increasing weight, elevated blood pressure and my LDL cholesterol was too high. After completing Dr Floyd's Detox/Cleansing program and "80% raw food" eating plan, I lost 14 lbs. My body fat % has declined, my blood pressure and pulse are at excellent levels. **More importantly, I feel great!! My energy level has increased dramatically and I feel great when I wake up every day!** I recommend this program to everyone – even those who "think" they are healthy!

Mary Jayne Maly
Houston, Texas

Dr. Floyd provided the information, encouragement and understanding to aid me in completing the cleansing program. Before the cleansing program I was tired a lot and needed a lot of rest to accomplish my work week. I had headaches and sinus problems often.

After the cleansing program, I am energized, have had few headaches or sinus problems and have learned to make new raw food dishes a staple of my diet .I really appreciate all of the help they have given me!

Annetta Allen
Houston, Texas

I would like to take the time to express my appreciation for the doctor and person you are. Your knowledge is great and anything you are not certain of, you thoroughly research and I am assured that it is the most updated information on the topic. During our Wellness Seminars your explanations are so clear it motivated everyone to take steps to improve their health.

You and your healing practices have helped me improve my eating habits and lose a total of 30 unwanted pounds.

As a doctor of Psychology, I have known you as a colleague and patient. When I refer a patient, I know they will be well cared for and will return physically healing in the mind, body, spirit process.

Willie Mae Lewis, PhD
Founder of Women's Resource Center of Houston

AN OUNCE OF

PREVENTION

A GUIDE TO LIVING IN A TOXIC WORLD

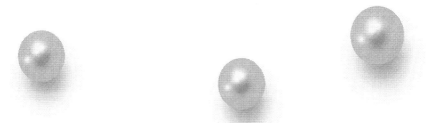

FIVE POWERFUL PEARLS THAT WILL

PRESERVE YOUR LIFE

by Dr. Floyd L. Atkins, Jr.

Center for Wellness and Healing Publishing
2002 Binz Street, Suite B
Houston, Texas 77004-7502

AN OUNCE OF PREVENTION

A Guide to Living in a Toxic World

Five Powerful Pearls That Will Preserve Your Life

By Dr. Floyd L. Atkins, Jr.

Publisher: Center for Wellness and Healing
2002 Binz Street, Suite B
Houston, Texas 77004-7502

Library of Congress Control Number: 2009907225
ISBN: 978-0-9841675-0-0

Printed in the United States of America.

First Edition, September 2009

Publisher's Note: This book is intended as a reference volume only, not as a medical manual. The ideas, suggestions and recommendations contained in this book are not intended as a substitute for consulting with your personal medical practitioner. Neither the publisher nor the author shall be liable or responsible for any loss or damage allegedly arising from any information or suggestions in this book. Furthermore, if you suspect you have a medical problem, we urge you to seek professional medical care.

The book may be bulk ordered at special rates.
Contact Dr. Floyd L. Atkins, Jr. @ drfloyd@drfloydatkins.com or write to Center for Wellness and Healing, 2002 Binz Street, Suite B, Houston, Texas 77004-7502.

ACKNOWLEDGMENTS

I would like to gratefully acknowledge the immeasurable support of my wife, Pamela Brewer Atkins, MD, for her constant encouragement to complete this book. Her knowledge, input and perspective has been an invaluable asset.

I must mention two others who have been a source of knowledge and inspiration: Maxine Murray, ND and Robert Young, PhD

I also want to recognize every patient and persons we have assisted over the years who have been the inspiration for me to continually dig deeper for answers. Each health challenge has been an opportunity for me to grow in "holistic" experience and knowledge and serve as a guide to those traveling on their "road to wellness."

DEDICATIONS

This book is dedicated first, to my mother and my father who put me on a

path of righteousness and gave me the tools I needed for this life.

To my sister, Edna, and brother, Edgar, who have been my lifelong trust and

support and finally, to each of my five sons and lovely daughter all of whom I

am most proud for they are my hope and my future.

About The Author

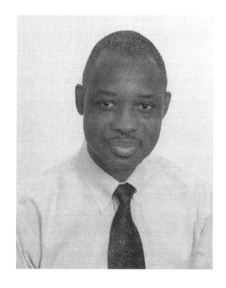

Dr. Floyd Atkins is a graduate of Morehouse College, BA in Biology 1975; a 1982 graduate of the Ohio College of Podiatric Medicine and completed his residency training at Kirwood General Hospital, Detroit, Michigan 1983. He was Board Certified in Foot Surgery in 1990 and is a lecturer and national speaker. He entered the ministry in 1996 and became an advocate for spiritual and physical wellness in the effort to connect the dots between mind, body, and spirit. Retiring from Podiatry in 2003, he pursues his passions in preventive health and wellness. The complement of high quality medical services and wellness education makes the vision of Drs. Pamela and Floyd Atkins' Center for Wellness and Healing a reality that is the cutting edge of a new and natural approach to healthcare.

CONTENTS

FOREWORD

In *An Ounce of Prevention*, Dr. Floyd Atkins shows the seeker of health how to RECLAIM Life; the good life. Rather than just survive an illness...we can THRIVE. We can actually heal. Open this book and you will find an abundance of information and guidance. You will learn: *How to prevent illness. How to heal.* And...*How to live a life that is Joyous, Happy & free!* Free of all physical dis-eases that harm us mentally, emotionally & spiritually.

Dr. Floyd stresses the importance of "good stewardship;" embracing the care of our mind, body & soul—wholistic healing. I've learned from him that I must value, minister to, & heal all three together. In a medical practice that has span over a period of more than 25-years Dr. Floyd has found that we, as a people, are "perishing," not from a lack of medication or surgery but from a lack of knowledge. This book supplies a solid a cure for that ailment.

He challenges us to STOP managing disease and to START healing through a life of *living wellness* that will prevent most occurrences of ill health.

Dr. Floyd teaches us that we can start today. He gives us, layman as well as interested physicians, fundamental prevention and intervention archetypes and models to follow. For example "Let food be thy medicine." Said, and advocated by Hippocrates centuries ago and by Dr. Floyd on today.

Dr. Floyd says we are still in control of our life, health, and well-being and that we must assume that responsibility. He does not just chide us, or lecture us, but in this book, shows us how. *An Ounce of Prevention*, well worth the pound of cure we will receive. I recommend it highly.

—Shirley Lundy-Connor M.Ed –Author, *How To Recover & Stay In Recovery* and *God's Promises-A Journal of Personal Growth & Discovery.*

PREFACE

♫ AWAKENING ♫

It was about Thanksgiving of 1974 when my "Return to Wellness" began. I was home from college and we were sitting in the living room after dinner laughing and reminiscing as was our normal family ritual. My mother pulled out a volume of our gray with red stripe, 4-volume medical encyclopedia, which was our consultant on any and all health issues and handed it to me. She casually said that she had felt a mass in her abdomen that had arisen since her summer physical exam. Mom continued saying she went to the doctor and he informed her that the mass was a grapefruit-sized tumor and a biopsy showed it to be cancer. I did not get too alarmed about her revelation since I knew of or had heard of very few people getting cancer and even fewer dying of the condition. While she was still speaking I began to read through that home medical encyclopedia only to discover that there was very little information about the causes or cure for cancer. As I left for college after that holiday, I continuously wondered where did the cancer come from and how it could be overcome. My somewhat desperate curiosity began that day and it remains undiminished until this day.

My mother was a well read, college-educated, spiritual and social activist in the community, a physically fit person, who had never been sick even with so much as a cold. Her battle with ovarian cancer, surgical intervention and the rough two series of radiation treatments devastated her body and she survived less than 18 months. In August 2005, nearly 30 years after my mother's death, my father succumbed to lung cancer after a brief illness. He did smoke cigarettes over 40 years of his life, although he stopped smoking more than 22 years before his death. He underwent several rounds of powerful chemotherapy, only for his doctors to tell him that the results were not positive. This experience was again confirmation for me that surgery, radiation, and chemotherapy were not a cure and also that virtually no real progress has been made in the fight against cancer.

After 25+ years of wondering how dis-eases such as cancer manifest, I experienced a spiritual revelation that was truly the answer to what was an apparent mystery. The absolute difference in the way our grand-relatives lived and the way we live today is our diet, our lifestyle, and our environmental exposures. Since the days of the original Eden, our body's ability to defend against disease has continuously declined and the toxic assault of our man-made environment has exponentially increased and continues to do so.

This book is written, not to accentuate the negatives of a world and healthcare system gone bad, but to inspire the readers to assume personal responsibility to Return to Wellness.

> [16] Don't you know that you yourselves are God's temple and that God's Spirit lives in you? [17] If anyone destroys God's temple, God will destroy him; for God's temple is sacred, and you are that temple. [18] Do not deceive yourselves. If any one of you thinks he is wise by the standards of this age, he should become a "fool" so that he may become wise.
>
> 1 Corinthians 3:16-18

INTRODUCTION

> *Insanity: doing the same thing over and over again and expecting different results.*
> *-   Albert Einstein*

∬ TIME TO CHANGE ∬

This book is written to change the way you look at your life in order to save your life. "An Ounce of Prevention" will not only provide the direction needed   to achieve optimal health, but also will present a roadmap of how to get there.

Let me share my background with you. I am a podiatrist completing my podiatric medical training and surgical residency in 1983, board certified in foot surgery in 1990 and operated an active surgical and Sport Medicine practice. I was well-trained and well respected in my profession.

I spent over 20 years in practice as a podiatric surgeon treating the symptoms of peoples' problems, trained in not addressing the root causes of problems, but basically skilled in eliminating symptoms. Once I had a patient that was a diabetic, with hypertension, and extremely poor circulation in her legs and multiple ulcers on her feet. She had been scheduled for an amputation and came to my office asking if there was anything I could do to save her leg. I immediately instituted an arsenal of wound care treatments to hopefully avoid the loss of her leg only to realize after several weeks, that with all my medical knowledge, training and technology, I had no real help to offer her. That's when it hit me… she did not need treatment, but "healing." That meant addressing the cause of her problem. Her problem was not the foot scheduled for amputation, but poorly controlled diabetes, poor diet, and lack of nutritional support. My patient was perishing from lack of knowledge, not lack of medication or surgery.

This was the beginning of my age of enlightenment understanding that health care was not about managing disease but healing, prevention, and wellness. Hippocrates (and Imhotep) said, "Let food be thy medicine," but today we must say, "Let natural (unprocessed), unmodified, locally-grown, organic food be thy medicine."

Answer these 5 questions honestly to determine where you are on your "Road to Wellness."

1). Do you still shop at a grocery where there is a healthy or natural foods section? (What is the quality of food in the rest of the store?)

2). Do you read and understand the ingredients of every food or product you put into your mouth or on your body?

3). How many grams of processed sugar do you eat or drink daily?

4). Do you participate in an hour or more of physical activity daily?

5). Do you pray, meditate or practice other stress-reduction techniques daily?

There are many more questions I could ask to determine where you are on "the Road," but most importantly, we must move forward from wherever we are.

The information to follow is presented to confirm that we are still in control of our life, health, and well-being. The challenge is that **we** must assume the responsibility to insure our prosperity…not our physician, our spouse, family or friends. Each and every day we must practice "good" stewardship over our mind, soul and body. We are the author and finisher of our fate on a day-to-day basis. The choices we make determine for us an abundant life or an untimely demise.

To achieve optimal health and wellness, we must live a life that not only helps others, but also "focuses attention" on ourselves - mind, soul, and body.

Attend to yourself. Ask, Seek and Knock!

PART ONE

THE PROBLEM

WARNING

Chemicals Known To The State Of
California To Cause Cancer, Or Birth
Defects Or Other Reproductive Harm
May Be Present In Foods Or Beverages
Sold Or Served Here.

LIVING IN A TOXIC WORLD

> *The blood, urine, and breast milk taken from*
> *72 adults identified the presence of 455*
> *chemicals that should <u>not</u> be in the body!*

∬ PRECARIOUS CIRCUMSTANCES ∬

Have you taken time to read the labels on the foods you eat? You definitely need a degree in biochemistry to understand what you are eating. We are engulfed in an invisible world of synthetic additives, preservatives, artificial colors and flavors, modified proteins and molecules that we largely ignore because we cannot see them. Most people have no realization of the quantities of these petroleum-based substances they ingest or the effects on their bodies. Reading the ingredient label on a Honey Bun seems more like a recipe for jet fuel than food for human consumption. Again, we give little thought to the side effects or after effects of eating such highly processed products.

The human body consists of billions of microscopic living cells, composed of perfectly, balanced quantities of water and organic substances. The biochemistry of the body can tolerate toxins only to a point, then, systems break down and disease sets in. Our generation like no other has become a giant experiment of toxic ingestion. We may consider our way of eating as normal, but the Standard American Diet (SAD) is about as normal as eating a test tube of chemicals.

Our body's chemistry is actually recreated by ingesting countless food additives and environmental contaminants. The toxins in our body have been accumulating since birth and are imbedded in every cell structure and organ. Toxins disrupt the natural chemistry of our body. Chemicals that have the power to produce mutations through chromosome damage cause disruptions of the genetic code. These mutagens are responsible for over 15,000 inheritable, genetic disorders that may have drastic consequences on us, our children and our grandchildren.

The food industry aim is to make products look and taste appealing without any consideration to the products' nutritional value. Processed foods are manufactured for profit, loaded with chemical additives and even designed to be addictive with additives such as high fructose corn syrup. Our bodies have become a chemical depository for sulfites used to keep dried fruit fresh, and formaldehyde used to disinfect frozen vegetables. The blue shimmer on the surface of luncheon meat is the result of sodium nitrate, a commonly used in the preservation of ham, bacon, sausage, and bologna. It is used to keep meat looking red, when normally it would have decomposed into an unappealing gray. In the stomach, sodium nitrate is converted into nitrous acid, which is suspected of being a prerequisite to stomach cancer. This powerful toxin is banned in Germany and Norway.

Lemon juice is widely used as a natural flavor enhancer for foods, but to cut cost and for convenience, manufacturers have replaced lemon juice with 2-methyl-3-(pisopropylphenyl)-propionaldehyde. This is just one of another estimated three thousand chemical additives we consume as a part of the American diet.

The life of most cells in our body is short and new cells are constantly being made to replace dead ones. The raw materials for this rebuilding come from what we eat, digest, and absorb into our blood stream. When it contains toxins, the process of rebuilding cells is disrupted. The basic biochemistry of

14

the body is compromised and our immunity to disease is diminished. If you have a genetic weakness and continue to eat processed foods, the cumulative effect of toxins will increase the risk of becoming a host to disease or premature death.

STATISTICS ON CHEMICAL EXPOSURE

Just how many chemicals are we exposed to on regular basis? The Environmental Working Group (EWG) reports that their ongoing monitoring project regularly tests. Finding two or three chemicals may not a big deal, but you must believe that as many as 455 can be harmful to the body.

Another recent EWG survey of some 2,300 Americans found that the average adult is exposed to 126 chemicals every day -- just in their personal care product use alone. One in every 13 women is exposed to a known or a probable human carcinogen every day with one in every 24 women, approximately 4.3 million, being exposed to personal care ingredients that are known or probable reproductive and developmental toxins. Could this be a direct environmental route from chemical exposure to breast cancer?

Women who use make-up on a daily basis can absorb almost 5 pounds of chemicals into their bodies each year. Some of the compounds present in make-up have been linked to side effects ranging from skin irritation to cancer. One class of cosmetic chemicals which are considered dangerous in Europe is parabens. Traces of parabens have been found in breast tumor samples.

Nine out of ten women also use out-of-date lipstick and mascara, which can be a breeding ground for harmful bacteria. Many women use more than 20 different beauty products a day and the effects of these multiple combinations of chemicals are for the most part unknown.

Researchers from the U.S. Centers for Disease Control and Prevention (CDC) have reported that 15 brands of powdered infant formula are contaminated with perchlorate, a rocket fuel component detected in drinking water in 28 states and territories.

The two most contaminated brands, made from cow's milk, accounted for 87 percent of the U.S. powdered formula market in 2000, the scientists said.

As early as the 1990's, a government study about toxic chemicals released by the Centers for Disease Control and Prevention (CDC) documents levels of more than 100 toxic chemicals found in the bodies of Americans. The CDC's study showed that the American public is exposed to a variety of chemicals, many of which have been linked to cancer, learning disabilities, or other chronic conditions like Parkinson's disease.

Here are some other startling results revealed by those findings:

ENVIRONMENTAL—

Pesticides and a host of other toxic chemicals have inundated our environment and pose possibly the most serious health hazard in today's world. Pesticides effects on humans are damaging to the nervous system, reproductive system and other organs. They result in developmental and behavioral abnormalities, immune dysfunction as well as disruption of hormone function.

Pesticides can be absorbed through the skin, swallowed or inhaled. According to the annual survey by U.S. Department of Agriculture (USDA) Pesticide Data Program, residues of organophosphate pesticides are routinely detected in food items commonly consumed by young children.

A study funded by the U.S. Environmental Protection Agency (EPA) and published in the September 2005 issue of Environmental Health Perspectives shows eating organic foods provides children with "dramatic and immediate" protection from exposure to two organophosphate pesticides that have been linked to harmful neurological effects in humans.

- Children have twice the levels of chlorpyrifos (Dursban) and other commonly used organophosphate insecticides as do adults.
- Mexican Americans have three times the levels of the pesticide DDT as do whites and blacks. DDT is a global contaminant that, while long banned in the US and more recently in Mexico, continues to be used against malaria in some countries.
- Levels of the chemicals called phthalates that are found in cosmetics are higher in adults, especially African American women, while the more toxic phthalates found in soft PVC plastic products are higher in children.

The latest and most pervasive assault on our health and wellness is Electromagnetic Fields (EMF). EMFs are invisible electrical and magnetic forces that radiate from anything operating on an electrical current. When any electrical current runs through a wire or an appliance, it produces an electromagnetic field.

Electromagnetic fields have long been associated with disease with the initial study done in 1979. Between 1985 and 1995, there have been 29 studies exploring the link to occupational EMF (e.g. electrical power linemen, telecommunication workers, electricians) with brain tumors incidence. One of these studies found an almost fourfold risk increase in brain tumors as compared to a non-exposed control group. Similarly, there are a significant number of adult leukemia studies that point to increased risk of leukemia with EMF exposures.

The frequencies at which cell phones emit EMFs are similar to those are emitted by a microwave oven. Therefore, placing a wireless phone next to your head is equivalent to heating your brain tissue with microwave radiation. Although the cell phone industry continues to claim that their products are safe, they also state on their product inserts that "there is no proof, however, that wireless phones are absolutely safe." In 1996, the FCC, working with the FDA, the US Environmental Protection Agency, and other agencies established RF (radio frequency) exposure safety guidelines for wireless phones in the U.S. One of these limits, Specific Absorption Rate or "SAR," is a measure of the rate of absorption of RF energy into the body. This radiation is not to exceed 1.6 watts per kilogram. Cell phones companies respond this way. "The actual SAR value of a wireless phone while operating can be less than the reported SAR value, but the SAR values may vary from call to call, depending upon the proximity to the cell tower, proximity to the body and the use of hand-free devices." In other words, there is no way to predict or guarantee exactly what amount RF exposure we actually receive, but it surely exceeds government limits.

Lastly, a study by UCLA Professor Leeka Kheifets found that pregnant moms who regularly used cell phones were much more likely to have a child who had emotional problems and hyperactivity by the time they reached school age. And children who used mobile phones themselves before the age of seven increased their risk of developing emotional problems by 80 percent.

CANCER—

Joel Fuhrman, MD in his article on "How to Win the War on Cancer" sums it up this way:

> We live in an era where the majority of Americans think that diseases strike us because of either, misfortune, genetics, or unknown factors beyond our control. When serious disease "strikes," we run to doctors and expect them to fix us with a pill. Most people have no idea that most diseases--including cancers, heart disease, strokes, and diabetes--are the result of nutritional

folly. Because they do not know whether adults lived longer centuries ago, they accept the myth that we are living healthier and longer today.

If we were taught from childhood that the diseases we suffer in the modern world are the tragic consequence of our toxic food environment, we wouldn't be in today's disgraceful situation--where people graduate from high school, college, and even graduate school without learning how to protect, preserve, and restore their precious health. With proper health education, we would learn that our bodies are powerfully resistant to disease when nutritional needs are met. Instead, we have become the victims of the high-tech, mass-produced food culture that is fueling a cancer epidemic unrivaled in human history.

Recent data on cancer statistics shows that we have gained very little ground over the last 40 years.

- One tenth of one percent of the U.S. budget is invested in cancer research.
- Cancer may affect people at all ages, even fetuses, but the risk for most varieties increases with age.
- Cancer causes about 13% of all deaths.
- According to the American Cancer Society, 7.6 million people died from cancer in the world during 2007.
- Nearly all cancers are caused by abnormalities in the genetic material of the transformed cells. These abnormalities may be due to the effects of carcinogens, such as tobacco smoke, radiation, chemicals, or infectious agents.
- Each day, more than 1,500 Americans die of cancer, the second leading cause of death in the US. It is responsible for one-fourth of all deaths in the US.
- Since 1990, about 16 million new cancer cases have been diagnosed.

- The cost of cancer to the economy was more than $150 billion annually in 2002. Within a decade, it is likely to exceed $200 billion. We invest just over $4 billion annually to cure cancer.
- If cancer were cured today, the economic value to the United States would exceed $46 trillion, more than the entire financial assets of the country.

In 1971, President Richard Nixon declared America's war on cancer, promising to end its toll within a decade. Each subsequent administration has reaffirmed this commitment, yet the number of cancer cases and deaths continue to grow.

The average American woman has a one in eight chance of developing breast cancer. In the U.S in 2004, approximately 117 women per 100,000 developed breast cancer. In Japan the figures were 22 of 100,000; in China 21 of 100,000; and in Korea 7 of 100,000.

In a systematic comparison of ingredients in 7,500 personal care products and the government's list of cancer-causing chemicals, the Environmental Working Group has found that one of every 100 products on the market lists on the label a known or probable human carcinogen.

Sixty-two products, one out of 120 products assessed, listed ingredients certified by government authorities as known or probable human carcinogens, including shampoos, lotions, foundations, and lip balms manufactured by Almay, Neutrogena, Grecian Formula, and others. The cancer-causing ingredients range from coal tar in shampoo to quartz crystals contained in powders and linked to lung cancer. Federal law does not prohibit the use of carcinogens in cosmetics.

NUTRITION—

Food security is the first and foremost concern when it comes to thriving in a toxic environment. Food security exists when all people, at all times, have physical and economic access to sufficient, safe and nutritious food to meet their dietary needs and food preferences for an active and healthy life. When we read headlines and get research data from around the world, we can easily understand that we are "food insecure" in many ways.

Salmonella, Listeria, melamine, E. coli are just a few of the many food contaminants found in our fruits, vegetables, meats, even pet foods and represent an ongoing health hazard we confront daily.

A wide range of pharmaceuticals that include antibiotics, sex hormones, and drugs used to treat epilepsy and depression, has been found to contaminate drinking water supplies of at least 41 million Americans. This was reported by the Associated Press National Investigation Team after a 5-month investigation recently released.

Jane Houlihan, EWG Vice President for Research said, "Environmental Working Group's (EWG) studies show that tap water across the U.S. is contaminated with many industrial chemicals, and now we know that millions of Americans are also drinking low-level mixtures of pharmaceuticals with every glass of water." "The health effect of this cocktail of chemicals and drugs hasn't been studied, but we are concerned about risks for infants and others who are vulnerable."

The bottled water industry promotes an image of purity, but comprehensive testing by research groups reveals a surprising array of chemical contaminants in many bottled water brand, including toxic byproducts of chlorination at levels no different than routinely found in tap water. Cancer-causing contaminants in bottled water purchased in 5 states (North Carolina,

California, Virginia, Delaware and Maryland) and the District of Columbia substantially exceeded the voluntary standards established by the bottled water industry.

When it comes to the American diet, one out of every 50 American adults are now extremely obese, or are 100 pounds or more overweight. This is a four-fold increase since the 1980s and is blamed primarily overeating and sedentary lifestyles. Under the current approach to health, disorders such as obesity, diabetes, high blood pressure, high cholesterol, cancers, autoimmune disorders, hyperactivity disorders and depression are now commonplace.

> *"At least one-third of all cancers are attributable to poor diet, physical inactivity, and overweight. Thus, if our goal of reducing cancer incidence by 25% in the United States by 2015 is to be reached, cancer prevention efforts must include strong programs for healthy eating and physical activity. Such programs will also help to reduce the incidence of many other chronic diseases."*
>
> *Dileep G. Bal, MD, MS, MPH*
> *Past President, American Cancer Society*

There is no question that the average American diet and lifestyle greatly increase our risk of developing many kinds of disease. Diets high in animal protein and fats (red meat, poultry, dairy), processed foods, sugar and alcohol and low in fresh fruits, vegetables, whole grains, essential fats and legumes lead to a myriad of health problems. Our heavy consumption of animal fat and protein put us at greater risk for hormone-based cancers.

Quote:

"Consumers believe that 'if it's on the market, it can't hurt me.' And this belief is sometimes wrong". –

Director of FDA's Office of Cosmetics and Colors (FDA 1998)

PART TWO

THE SOLUTION

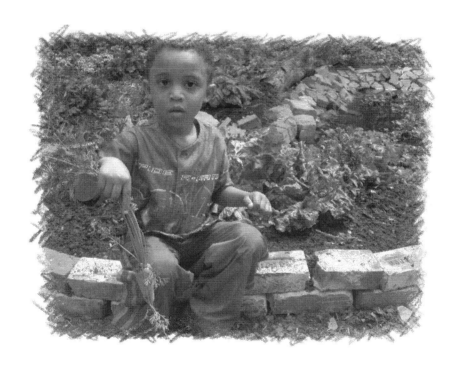

PREVENTION IS THE KEY

> *If cancer were cured today, the economic value to the United States would exceed 46 trillion dollars, more than the entire financial assets of our country.*

∫∫ TRANSFORMING OUR APPROACH TO HEALTHCARE ∫∫

How many times have we heard news and statistics about the increasing rate of illness and disease such as diabetes, high blood pressure, heart disease, cancer, arthritis and so on? News reports appear on television and radio daily about "new treatments" to reduce or eliminate symptoms. Billions of dollars are raised and spent on finding the cure for cancer, diabetes and the many other chronic ailments that plague us. Meanwhile, the rates of all these conditions have steadily increased over the last 50 years and still no "cures" have been found.

Since medical research seems unable to find cures for our most serious conditions, the "Plan B" solution in healthcare has become "early detection," as if it were the answer to our health challenges. This concept has credence, but waiting for or allowing a problem such as cancer to develop and then, to attempt to "catch it early" is not the most desirable goal. Although our efforts to stem the tide of disease are made with the best of intentions, our approach is all wrong!

Prevention is the answer! The true or absolute "cure" for all "dis-ease" is <u>not</u> to get it. I am sure this sounds over-simplified, but let's look at our healthcare history so we can understand our future in wellness.

The foundation of our current healthcare system is built upon the concept of the ER (emergency room), which is essential for saving lives in critical situations. The emergency room's original purpose was to address trauma or physical injuries to our bodies, mainly secondary to accidents. But today, it has become the catchall for almost of our health needs, major and minor. We have subtly programmed ourselves not even **to** think about our own health unless an emergency arises! Should you wait until your car stops on the side of the road to consider taking it in for maintenance? Would you wait to have a flat tire then check your tire for air pressure? Most people know more about their finances, stocks and FICA score than they do about their triglycerides, kidney or immune function.

Our approach to healthcare should be about prevention first. It sounds so common sense, but most people do not understand what prevention truly is. Many think that getting regular exercise and eating 5 to 9 fruits and vegetables daily is prevention. Prevention in the primary medical sense means "to avoid the development of dis-ease" and secondarily, "to stop the progression of a disease <u>before</u> symptoms arise." PREVENTION IS THE CURE TO DIS-EASE! Prevention is neither practiced nor promoted because we lack knowledge about ourselves and overlook wisdom in the way we live.

Let's look at the biblical basis for prevention as our key to optimal health. One only has to consider Hosea 4: 6 - "My people are destroyed for lack of knowledge." From the prospective of health and wellness, the scripture states that we are destroyed or "de-structured," i.e., broken down and taken apart bit by bit. Our bodies are being worn down daily because we do not know how to protect or preserve ourselves. The scripture further states this is not intentional, but because we lack knowledge or simply do not know. The converse of this scripture is that we are "re-structured or restored" with sufficiency of knowledge. Therefore, when we have knowledge and exercise wisdom, we can be restored with abundance. The scripture is also very clear that we have been already given everything we have need of, so where do we begin.

KNOWLEDGE

Populations that have a high intake of natural, unrefined plant foods such as fruits, vegetables, seeds, nuts, and beans always have a low incidence of cancer, proportional to the intake of these phytochemical-rich plant foods. Even though other factors such as chemicals, pollution, and smoking play a role in cause of cancer, scientific literature still illustrates that a better diet offers dramatic protection against cancer and most all chronic diseases.

Here is an example: An ecological study of diet and lung cancer in the South Pacific. Int J Cancer 1995 Sep 27 was conducted in the Fiji Islands. Although smoking rates varied, they have a dramatically lower incidence of lung cancer than Hawaii where smoking rates are lower. This protection against lung cancer even in heavily smoking Fiji Islanders was shown to be the result of the high intake of green vegetables in Fiji.

The World Cancer Research Fund, after reviewing data from numerous epidemiological studies, concluded that there was convincing evidence that fruits and vegetables may reduce the risk of oral, esophageal, lung, stomach, colon, pancreatic, bladder, and breast cancer. There was no single substance in a plant-based diet that accounts for this relationship, but rather, the synergistic effect of multiple phytochemical compounds.

In 2000, The National Cancer Institute recommended eating 5 servings of fruits and vegetables each day. However, scientific studies suggest that more is better and that much more is much, much better at reducing cancer risk.

Here is the latest update by NCI in 2005:

People whose diets are rich in plant foods such as fruits and vegetables have a lower risk of getting cancers of the mouth, pharynx, larynx, esophagus, stomach, lung, and there is some suggested evidence for colon, pancreas, and prostate. They are also less likely to get diabetes, heart disease, and hypertension. A diet high in fruits and vegetables helps to reduce calorie intake and may help to control weight.

To help prevent these cancers and other chronic diseases, experts recommend **4 to 13 servings of fruits and vegetables daily**, depending on energy needs. This includes 2 to 5 servings of fruits and 2 to 8 servings of vegetables, **with special emphasis on dark-green and orange vegetables and legumes**. There is no evidence that the popular white potato protects against cancer. Additional servings of fruits and vegetables should replace sources of "empty calories" in the diet, such as added sugars (honey, syrup, soft drinks) and solid fats (butter, sour cream), to avoid taking in too many calories.

Even more recent data has been reported concerning, the significance of prevention as the answer to our national and global health crisis. Carefully read this report that offers data and solutions.

For Immediate Release: 6:00 a.m. ET, Thursday, February 26th, 2009

Many Cancers Could Be Prevented
In the US and Across the Globe

Comprehensive, Evidence-Based Recommendations for All Levels of Society

WASHINGTON, DC – A new global policy report estimates that approximately **45 percent of colon cancer cases** and **38 percent of breast cancer cases** in the US are preventable through diet, physical activity and weight maintenance. The report also sets out recommendations for policies to reduce the global number of cancer cases.

The overall message of the report, *Policy and Action for Cancer Prevention*, published today by World Cancer Research Fund (WCRF) and American Institute for Cancer Research (AICR), is that all sections of society need to make public health and cancer prevention in particular, a higher priority.

It includes estimates on the proportion of many different types of cancer that could be prevented through diet, physical activity and weight management. **In the US, about one third of the most common cancers could be prevented**. That figure does not include smoking, which alone accounts for about a third of cancers.

Policy Report Represents the Next Step

The new WCRF/AICR Policy Report is a companion document to the expert report *Food, Nutrition, Physical Activity and the Prevention of Cancer: A Global Perspective*, which was published by AICR and WCRF in November of 2007. That expert report evaluated the scientific evidence from over 7000 studies and came away with 10 recommendations for lowering cancer risk.

"The 2007 expert report identified the specific choices that people can make to protect themselves against cancer, but actually making those healthy choices remains difficult for many people," said policy report panel member Shiriki Kumanyika, PhD, MPH, of the University of Pennsylvania School of Medicine. "The policy report takes the next step – it identifies opportunities for us as a society to make those choices easier."

PERCENTAGE OF CANCERS THAT COULD BE PREVENTED VIA HEALTHY DIET, REGULAR PHYSICAL ACTIVITY AND HEALTHY WEIGHT

	US	UK	Brazil	China
Endometrium (lining of the uterus)	70	56	52	34
Esophagus	69	75	60	44
Mouth, pharynx & larynx	63	67	63	44
Stomach	47	45	41	33
Colon	45	43	37	17
Pancreas	39	41	34	14
Breast	38	42	28	20
Lung	36	33	36	38
Kidney	24	19	13	8
Gallbladder	21	16	10	6
Liver	15	17	6	6
Prostate	11	20	n/a	n/a
These 12 cancers combined	**34**	**39**	**30**	**27**

***The American Institute for Cancer Research (AICR) is the cancer charity that fosters research on the relationship of nutrition, physical activity and weight management to cancer risk, interprets the scientific literature and educates the public about the results. AICR has published two landmark reports that interpret the accumulated research in the field, and is committed to a process of continuous review.

As part of the evidence-based report, thought to be the most comprehensive ever published on the subject, two independent teams of scientists systematically examined the evidence for how policy changes can influence the behaviors that affect cancer risk.

Following this, a panel of 23 world-renowned experts made a total of **48 recommendations**, divided between nine different but often overlapping sectors of society – called "actor groups" in the report. These actor groups are: multinational bodies; civil society organizations; government; industry; media; schools; workplaces and institutions; health and other professionals; and people.

Among the recommendations:

- **Governments** should require widespread **walking and cycling routes** to encourage physical activity.
- **Industry** should give a higher priority for goods and services that **encourage people to be active**, particularly young people.
- The **food and drinks industry** should make public health an explicit priority at all stages of production.
- **Schools** should actively encourage physical activity and provide healthy food for children.
- **Schools, workplaces and institutions** should not have unhealthy foods available in **vending machines**.
- **Health professionals** should take a lead in giving the public information about public health, including cancer prevention.
- **People** should use independent nutrition guides and food labels to make sure the food they buy for their family is healthy.

Based upon the continuously mounting body of evidence, a proactive prevention program is the Key and ultimate cure to disease.

I want to share with you "FIVE POWERFUL PEARLS OF PREVENTION." I consider these to be the 5 most important changes one can implement to prevent disease and reverse illness. It only takes an "Ounce of Prevention" to effect a "Pound of Cure." By incorporating these health practices and principles into your daily activities, you are not only changing lifestyle, but changing your approach to how you manage your health!

PART THREE

THE FIVE PEARLS OF PREVENTION

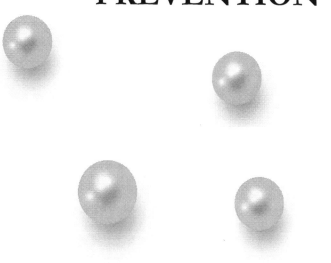

PEARL NUMBER ONE

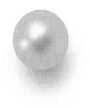

ʃʃ DETOXIFY, DON'T DIE ʃʃ

Toxic chemicals, both naturally occurring and man-made, often get into the human body. We may inhale them, swallow them in contaminated food or water, or in some cases, absorb them through skin. A woman who is pregnant may pass them to her developing fetus through the placenta. The term **"toxic burden"** refers to the total amount of these chemicals that are present in the human body at a given moment. Sometimes it is also useful to consider the toxic burden of a specific, single chemical, like, for example, lead, mercury, or dioxin.

Some chemicals or their breakdown products (metabolites) lodge in our bodies for only a short while before being excreted, but continuous exposure to such chemicals can create a "persistent" toxic burden. Arsenic, for example, is mostly excreted within 72 hours of exposure. Other chemicals, however, are not readily excreted and can remain for years in our blood, adipose (fat) tissue, semen, muscle, bone, brain tissue, or other organs. Chlorinated pesticides, such as DDT, can remain in the body for 50 years. Whether chemicals are quickly passing through or are stored in our bodies, toxic burden testing can reveal to us an individual's unique chemical load and can highlight the kinds of chemicals we are exposed to as we live out each day of our lives. Of the approximately 80,000 chemicals that are used in the United States, we do not know how many can become a part of our chemical toxic burden, but we do know that several hundred of these chemicals have been measured in people's bodies around the world.

Before we proceed, take a toxicity test that follows to get some idea of how toxicity may translate into physical signs and symptoms. This test should be repeated after you have completed one or more cleansing programs.

TOXICITY TEST

Do You Need A Cleanse?   **What's In Your Body?**   **Y / N**

1. Do you experience fatigue or low energy levels?   _____
2. Do you experience brain fog, lack of concentration and/or poor memory?   _____
3. Do you eat fast foods, fatty foods, pre-prepared foods, or fried foods?   _____
4. Do you drink coffee and sodas during the day to "get you going"?   _____
5. Do you smoke cigarettes?   _____
6. Do you crave or eat sugary snacks and candy or desserts?   _____
7. Do you have less than 2 bowel movements per day?   _____
8. Do you feel sleepy after meals, bloated and/or gassy?   _____
9. Do you experience indigestion after eating?   _____
10. Are you overweight or do you rarely exercise?   _____
11. Do you experience frequent headaches?   _____
12. Do you experience reoccurring yeast infections?   _____
13. Do you have arthritic aches and pains or stiffness?   _____
14. Do you take any prescription medication, sedatives, or stimulants?   _____
15. Do you live with or near polluted air, water or other environmental pollution? _____
16. Do you have bad breath or excessive body odor?   _____
17. Have you been told your cholesterol is elevated?   _____
18. Do you have high blood pressure or have BP that is elevated at times?   _____
19. Do you have recurrent sinus congestion or environmental symptoms?   _____
20. Do you experience depression or mood swings? (mental highs and lows)   _____
21. Do you have food allergies or bad skin?   _____
22. Are you showing signs of premature aging?   _____
23. Have you ever used an internal cleansing product and followed   _____
a complete internal cleansing program?

If you answered "yes" to 3 or more of the above-listed questions or answered "no" to question 20, you are a good candidate for an internal cleansing program and would benefit greatly. Cleansing programs detoxifies the organs of the body, helps to control weight, encourages the production of energy, and helps individuals feel more alive and healthy.

HOW WE BECOME TOXIC

Here is a list of the 8 most common causes of toxic build-up in the human body. This information can be a huge help in keeping you on a healthy path in life. Learn these basics and apply them to your everyday life by making the right choices...

1. CONSTIPATION - The colon is your body's sewage system. If your sewage system backs up, toxins become trapped in your colon. Chronic constipation means these toxins are fermenting and decaying in the colon, often being re-absorbed into the bloodstream, which in turn, pollutes all of our tissues and cells, and sets the stage for chronic disease and illness to follow.

2. POOR DIET - Poor diet includes dead, cooked, devitalized, clogging, low fiber foods, fried foods, junk foods, over-processed foods, etc. As a modern society, we have drifted further and further away from eating raw, organic "good for you" fruits, vegetables and whole grains high in natural fiber, nutrients, and enzymes. We now use processed and pre-prepared foods to fit with our busy lifestyles. Unfortunately these foods do nothing to benefit our health. These foods, unlike live foods (fresh, raw fruits and vegetables), lack the proper enzymes to assist in proper digestion and assimilation, and lack the fiber or bulk to assist in proper elimination. They are also lacking in essential vitamins, minerals and other basic, life giving nutrients.

3. OVER-CONSUMPTION - Overeating puts a tremendous amount of stress on our digestive system. Most people eat too much food, too fast. A meal should be eaten slowly and food chewed thoroughly. Saliva mixed with food in the mouth plays a huge role in foods being digested properly. The body must produce hydrochloric acid, pancreatic enzymes, bile and other digestive factors to process a meal. When we over-eat, the digestive system cannot always meet the demands placed upon it. The stomach bloats as the digestive system goes into turmoil. Foods are not properly broken down and tend to lodge in the lower intestines. Vital nutrients are NOT absorbed. Try to eat smaller meals, with "healthy" snacks in-between meals. If you only eat when you're "starving," you will constantly over-eat and wonder why you feel so heavy, bloated and tired afterwards.

4. LACK OF WATER - Water makes up 65 to 75% of the human body. It is second only to oxygen in order of importance to sustain life. Water cleanses the inside of the body as well as the outside. It is instrumental in flushing out wastes and toxins. When our bodies do not receive enough water, toxins tend to stagnate, hindering all digestive and eliminative processes. Drinking approximately one-half your weight in ounces of water a day is ideal for good health. By the way, sodas DO NOT COUNT as water intake! Sodas of any kind (Coke, Diet Coke, Sprite, etc.) contain high levels of sodium, sweeteners, caffeine, and very bad-for-you chemicals. Over time, sodas can be a big contributor to ill health.

5. STRESS - Stress affects every cell and tissue in the human body. Stress breaks down the immune system as well as all of the major organs. Have you ever noticed how much easier it is to get sick when you're under a lot of stress? Stress is TOXIC to our bodies! It robs the body of important vitamins and minerals, and over time, can cause severe acid build-up. Stress hinders proper digestion, absorption and elimination of foods by throwing the digestive system out of balance. The worst thing a person can do is to eat a meal while experiencing extreme stress. This usually causes indigestion, and nutrients will not be absorbed. Regulate and control the amount of stress in your life, and you will be a healthier and happier person.

6. ANTIBIOTICS - Antibiotics, despite their benefits in fighting certain bacterial infections, have a damaging effect on the intestines. Their prescribed purpose is to eliminate unhealthy bacteria in the body; bacteria that causes illness. However, antibiotics also eliminate the healthy, necessary, good bacteria in our bodies! They strip the colon of ALL intestinal flora...good and bad. After antibiotics are taken, it is usually the bad bacteria that regenerate and multiply quickly, often causing nagging yeast infections and digestive and eliminative upset. Our entire gastrointestinal tract becomes imbalanced, creating problems in the colon and hampering proper digestion. When we are forced to take antibiotics, it is extremely important to supplement our diets with cultured foods (yogurt and cottage cheese from organic sources) that contain live "good" bacteria, and probiotic supplements, preferably soiled-based organisms (SBOs). We must replace the good bacteria, for optimum health and proper intestinal function.

7. LACK OF EXERCISE - Exercise strengthens our entire bodies. It stimulates the circulatory and lymphatic system, building muscles, nerves, blood, glands, lungs, heart, brain, mind and mood. Blood is pumped throughout our bodies by the heart, but lymphatic fluid depends solely on exercise to be circulated throughout our lymphatic system. The lymphatic system is the human body's sewage system... it is responsible for the removal of cellular and toxic waste. Here is a remarkable fact... there is 3 times more lymphatic fluid in the human body than blood! Physical exercise and movement is the lymphatic system's only "pump," so to speak. If we don't exercise, our lymphatic system becomes sluggish and toxic, affecting our over-all health. Lack of exercise lowers metabolic efficiency, and without circulatory and lymphatic stimulation, the body's natural cleansing systems are weakened.

8. EATING LATE AT NIGHT - The human body uses sleep to repair, rebuild and restore itself. In essence, our bodies use the sleeping hours to cleanse and detoxify, and to build strength and immunity. When we eat late at night and go to sleep with a full stomach, the body IS NOT at rest. Even though our mental processes are quiet, our physical body is actually quite busy digesting and processing a large amount of food. This inhibits the vital cleansing, building and restorative processes that normally occur while we sleep. We've all had the experience of going to sleep with a full stomach, and waking the next morning feeling tired, exhausted and disoriented, despite 8 hours of sleep. This is because your body, in actuality, did NOT get 8 hours of sleep... more like 3 hours of sleep, after working hard most of the night to digest and process the big meal you ate before bed. Do not eat late at night! Eat an early dinner, and eat light in the evenings.

Undertaking a detoxification program requires a willingness to change, discipline to stay the course throughout the process, and a commitment to maintain the successes you have accomplished. The process may seem uncomfortable at times, but believe me; the options are much less desirable.

Here are summaries of the most effective detoxification methods for persons whose goal is to achieve optimal health or overcome a serious health challenge.

INTERNAL DETOXIFICATION

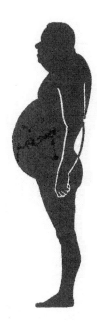

Most degenerative conditions have their origin in the malfunction of the digestive and liver detoxification processes. In other words, illness can be directly related to problems of the digestive and liver detoxification systems and their related influence on immune, nervous and endocrine function. Therefore, if we address the health of these systems, the body is given the opportunity to create foundational health throughout the rest of the body. Whether a degenerative condition is labeled lupus, diabetes, arthritis, or any other "condition," addressing the health of the digestive tract is recommend. Once the GI tract is clear, then the liver detoxification system should be supported and strengthened.

3 key points about cleansing:

❖ Address the health of the gastrointestinal tract first, no matter what the name of the degenerative disease, simply because the dynamics of the body make it clear that conditions in the digestive tract affect the entire system.

❖ The breakdown of the gastrointestinal environment is one of the primary points at which health is lost. What we now know is that the same toxins associated with GI dysfunction are frequently absorbed and distributed to other parts of the body.

❖ Toxic burden is placed on the liver and the immune system first. If liver overload occurs, there will be spillover, and some of the toxins will be passed on to other organs or tissues.

PRIMARY DETOXIFICATION METHODS

There are many different ways to detoxify depending upon what specific health issues you wish to address, what goal you wish to accomplish or the level of cleansing your body is able to tolerate.

There are:

1. Herbal-based detox program which usually place emphasis on the colon cleansing and parasite elimination;
2. Natural mineral chelation-like detox/cleanse- this is a toxin-specific cleanse that targets heavy metals, pesticides, herbicides, and other positively charged toxins from the system. A naturally occurring, negatively charged mineral called Zeolite is formed from the fusion of volcanic lava and ocean water and is an extremely effective detoxifier.

3. FIR saunas, sweat lodges and bath soaks- these are designed for persons to release toxins through their skin rather than via organs, e.g., kidney, liver and colon. This is especially important for those individuals who have compromised liver, kidney or colon function and cannot tolerate additional burden on those organs.

4. Fasting-type programs which are usually associated with goals toward weight loss, i.e., juice fasting, lemonade fast, etc.

HERBAL DETOXIFICATION

An herbal detoxification program utilizes herbs at therapeutic dosages to cleanse, repair, and rebuild damaged tissues and organs. A thorough and complete herbal detox program should include:

- a colon and kidney cleanse
- a parasite cleanse and heavy metal detox
- A liver/gall bladder cleanse at minimum.

There should also be a significant dietary change in order not to re-pollute our body with the same toxic, devitalized food we just cleansed out. This food eating program should support the herbal detoxification by incorporating primarily whole food nutrition. This means that your diet during the cleansing period should eliminate all processed foods (anything in cans, cartons, plastics, or frozen) and include an 80% organic raw food menu with spring water. All "white foods" (white flour, white sugar, white potatoes and white rice) should be eliminated as well as all red meat and caffeinated/carbonated beverages.

By detoxifying and cleansing, we can eliminate:

1) mucoid plaque from your digestive tract,
2) multiple parasites from digestive tract and organs,
3) gallstones and toxic debris from your liver, and finally,

45

4) It will support and repair damaged organ systems.

Detoxifying and cleansing of your internal environment is the foundation of optimal health, wellness and longevity. An overloaded congested colon, parasites, gallstones and toxic debris all interfere with our body's ability to function properly as well as severely hampers our immune system.

The changes that may be seen from detoxifying and cleansing are:

- lower total and "LDL" cholesterol levels
- reduced blood pressure
- shedding pounds and reduced body fat
- better blood sugar control
- reduction in allergy symptoms
- increase overall energy
- increase mental alertness
- greater sense of well-being

The goal of a detoxification program is to cleanse and reduce the toxic burden on your internal organs thereby assisting in restoring metabolic balance. Additionally, the amount of toxins stored in body fat is dramatically reduced paving the way for an increased ability to burn excess fat.

We medically supervise a 6-Week Detox/Cleanse Program and our results have been beyond remarkable. We have compared before and after laboratory results of patients to measure their change or success.

Here are some typical results from two patients who completed the program:

Detox/Cleanse Program Results

050747AR-57yo male

	Before	After	Reference Values
Date	12/23/2003	04/08/2004	
Triglycerides	399	62	<150 mg/dl
Cholesterol, Total	261	174	<200 mg/dl
HDL	49	53	> or =40 mg/dl
LDL	132	109	<130 mg/dl
Hemoglobin A1C	10.2%	5.9%	<6.0% (non-diabetic)
Blood Pressure	138/92	120/88	
Pulse	74	60	
Weight	197	192	
Body Fat Index	26.1%	24.8%	<25%
Body Fat Mass	51 lbs	47 lbs	

Detox/Cleanse Program Results

B43051JR-54yo male

	Before	After	Reference Values
Date	02/08/2005	04/08/2005	
Triglycerides	234	123	<150 mg/dl
Cholesterol, Total	172	124	<200 mg/dl
HDL	35	36	> or =40 mg/dl
LDL	90	63	<130 mg/dl
Hemoglobin A1C	6.0%	5.4%	<6.0% (non-diabetic)
Blood Pressure	150/98	120/80	
Pulse		58	
Weight	220	202	
Body Fat Index	29.7%	26.6%	<25%
Body Fat Mass	63 lbs	54 lbs	

MINERAL CHELATION DETOXIFICATION

As many as 25 percent of Americans are estimated to suffer from some degree of heavy metal poisoning, particularly from mercury, lead, cadmium, and arsenic. According to the EPA, 70,000 chemicals are used commercially in the U.S., 65,000 of which are potentially hazardous to our health. The Environmental Defense Council reports that more than four billion pounds of toxic chemicals are released into the environment each year, including 72 million pounds of known carcinogens.

A joint study by Mt. Sinai School of Medicine, Commonwealth, and the Environmental Working Group in 2003 identified a total of 167 hazardous compounds in the blood and urine of American adults (with an average of 91 per person tested), including 76 known to cause cancer, 94 that are toxic to the nervous system, 82 that damage the lungs, 86 that affect hormone function, and 79 that cause birth defects.

Zeolite, a naturally occurring, negatively charged mineral, with a unique crystalline structure is formed from the fusion of volcanic lava and ocean water. It has been used for 800 years throughout Asia as a traditional remedy to promote overall health and well-being and for 30 years in the U.S. in animal feed. It has also undergone 13 years of pharmaceutical research in the U.S. with humans. Zeolite is included on the Food and Drug Administration's GRAS list (generally recognized as safe) and thus is considered to be "completely safe."

Zeolite is probably the most effective, single natural substances for removing a broad range of chemical and viral toxins from the body with virtually no risk. Because it neutralizes toxic chemicals on contact, there is no subsequent "detoxification or Herxheimer reaction" occurrence as they are eliminated.

Zeolite clinoptilolite is an insoluble rock crystal. A micronizing process is used in order to make the rock particle small (a few microns in size) so they can be absorbed into the body via the intestines.

Clinoptilolite has been the subject of a large number of studies in regard to its established ability to bind toxic metals. In a few laboratory studies on various cancer cell cultures and tumor-bearing animals, zeolite clinoptilolite prolonged life and in some cases reduced tumor size. Scientific studies of mice and dogs showed improvement in their overall health, life extension and reduction in tumor sizes. Local application to dogs' skin cancers also exhibited a reduction in both tumor formation and growth.

MEDICAL BENEFITS OF ZEOLITE

G. I. Benefits

- anti-diarrheal product: best known positive activity (prescription: Enterex)
- has high affinity for ammonium ions in G.I. tract
- aids the buffering capacity of G.I. secretions (pH buffering)
- has positive effect on bacterial flora and the re-absorption of vitamins & minerals
- has been used successful as a treatment for both diarrhea and IBS

Binding Capabilities

- binds mycotoxins that can cause renal & hepatic symptoms and decreases immune function
- binds/absorbs aflatoxins (linked to liver, stomach & kidney cancers); (2 studies 1992/2002)

- has high affinity for trapping lead, cadmium, arsenic, mercury & other harmful metals
- decreases overall metal exposure in individuals reducing risk of certain cancers and heart disease
- tendency to bind/remove heavy metals first, then the secondary toxins, i.e., pesticides, herbicides, & plastics

Anti-Oxidant Activity

- Has capacity to trap free radicals into its structure, thereby inactivating and eliminating them; in contrast to traditional antioxidants which neutralizes by absorbing excess free radicals.

Cancer Prevention

- traps carcinogens such as nitrosamines found specifically in processed meats, beer & cigarette smoke
- presence of zeolite inside a cancer cell activates the p21 gene which suppresses tumor growth

Anti-Viral Activity

- zeolite traps pre-viral components preventing the reduction of viruses
- able to block development of many viral infections including Herpes I
- case studies show Herpes zoster become pain free within 1-3 days after taking zeolite
- shown effective in treating flu, colds and Hepatitis C
- shown effective in treating mral or heavy metal induced MS & RA
- helps liver enzymes (AST & ALT) return to normal levels

Immune Support

- Zeolite helps balance the immune system by effectively removing toxins which increase energy, well being and mental clarity.

Zeolite when taken over a 4 to 8 week period

- ❖ tends to eliminate pesticides and herbicides in the first 3-4 weeks,
- ❖ then begin its anti-viral action

Zeolite is commercially available in a purified and activated form. There are no reports of side effects, except one: because of its natural action to absorb water, zeolite can cause dehydration. It is therefore important to drink sufficient water (approximately one-half your weight in ounces) both before and while taking zeolite to ensure adequate hydration.

Since zeolite is an insoluble crystalline structure, it technically cannot maintain its structure or properties if converted into a liquid form. For this reason, only a solid form in powder or capsule is recommended.

There is only one contraindication: **Zeolite is contraindicated for anyone taking a medication containing heavy metals, such as lithium, or containing platinum, which is found in some cancer medications.** Before taking Zeolite, check with your doctor to determine if your medication contains heavy metals or platinum.

HYPERTHERMIC DETOXIFICATION

FAR INFRARED SAUNA (FIR)

Saunas and steam baths have been used for centuries by cultures around the world to bring about detoxification. Traditionally, saunas have been used to improve mental clarity, to diminish pain and promote longevity. In the past few years, hyperthermic (sweat) therapy has been studied quite extensively and several papers on this subject have appeared in the scientific literature. Through this research, it has been shown that saunas greatly assist in the elimination of accumulated toxins. Toxic metals, including mercury as well as organic toxins such as PCB's and pesticide residues, are excreted in high quantities in the sweat during properly conducted hyperthermic therapy sessions.

Heat causes toxins to be released from cells. The toxic molecules will then reside transiently in the lymph fluid. Since sweat is manufactured from the lymph fluid, toxins present in the lymph fluid will exit the body through the sweat. Because the liver and kidneys are not required for this process, these organs are largely unburdened by hyperthermic therapy and toxins are able to leave the body even when liver or kidney function is impaired. This may be a distinct advantage for chronically ill patients whose livers and kidneys may already be under toxic stress.

ADVANTAGES OF FAR INFRARED SAUNA

In these traditional systems, the inside of the body is heated completely from the surface of the skin. Even though you feel very hot in these units, the heating is quite shallow - only a few millimeters below the skin. In the far infrared sauna, invisible light rays emanate from several infrared emitters. This infrared light penetrates deep into the fat and muscles of the body, creating a more powerful detoxifying influence upon the deeper tissues of the body. Also, since the air temperature remains much lower than in a traditional sauna, the individual feels more comfortable. Sweating often begins before the person feels very hot at all and the sweating is more profuse than in a traditional sauna.

In Guyton's **Textbook of Medical Physiology**, we find that producing one gram of sweat requires 0.586 kcal (586 calories).

As reported in the Journal of the American Medical Association (JAMA), August 7, 1981, "A moderately conditioned person can easily sweat off 500 gms. in a sauna, consuming nearly 300 kcal - the equivalent of running 2 - 3 miles. A heat-conditioned person can easily sweat off 600 - 800 kcal with no adverse effects. <u>While the weight of the water loss can be regained by rehydration with water, **the calories consumed will not be**</u>."

Since an infrared sauna helps generate two to three times the sweat produced in a hot-air sauna, the implications for increased caloric consumption are quite impressive.

Calories a 150-pound person normally burns up in 30-minutes of exercise:

SPORTS	CALORIES
Marathon Running	593
Vigorous Racquet Ball	510
Swimming (freestyle)	300
Jogging	300
Tennis (fast game)	265
Cycling (10 mpg)	225
Golfing (without a cart)	150
Walking (3.5 mph)	150
Bowling	100

The JAMA citation referred to above goes on to state that, "Many of us who run do so to place a demand on our cardiovascular system, not to build big leg muscles. Regular use of a sauna may impart a similar stress on the cardiovascular system, and its regular use may be as effective, as a means of cardiovascular conditioning and burning of calories, as regular exercise."

OTHER ADVANTAGES OF HYPERTHERMIA THERAPY

Hyperthermic therapy is one of the few therapies which stimulate a significant rise in the level of growth hormone, an important hormone that helps to maintain lean body tissue, including muscle.

Hyperthermic therapy helps to restore normal autonomic nervous system functioning. Autonomic dysregulation is the term used to describe changes in the nervous system, which result in many of the symptoms of chronic fatigue and fibromyalgia. This is the part of the nervous system is responsible for unconscious functions such as blood pressure, digestion, muscle tension, sweating and balance. Some of the many manifestations of autonomic dysregulation are:

- Muscle pain
- excessive body odor
- digestive complaints
- visual disturbances and
- dizziness

Repeated sessions of hyperthermic therapy can greatly assist in the restoration of normal autonomic nervous system functioning.

BENEFITS OF THE FAR INFRARED SAUNA

Robert O. Young, PhD in his book, *Sick and Tired? Reclaim Your Inner Terrain,* revealed the results of two years of his research on radiant heat (infrared) sauna which showed the following benefits:

- ✓ Speeds up metabolic processes of vital organs and glands, including endocrine glands.
- ✓ Inhibits the development of pleomorphic microforms (fungi, yeasts and bacteria) and creates a "fever reaction" of rising temperature that neutralizes them.
- ✓ Increases the number of leukocytes in the blood
- ✓ Places demand on the heart to work harder thus, exercising it and also producing a drop in diastolic blood pressure (the low side)
- ✓ Stimulates dilation of peripheral blood vessels thus, relieving pain (including muscle pain) and speeding the healing of sprain, strain, bursitis, arthritis, and peripheral vascular disease symptoms
- ✓ Promotes relaxation thereby creating a feeling of well-being.

For those who are unable to exercise sufficiently, for whatever reason, the radiant heat infrared sauna is an excellent way to get the benefits of exercise without undue stress on the skeleton, muscles, and associated tissues. Such people have an even greater need for exercise and the sauna fills the bill.

Finally, unlike traditional saunas or steam baths, which can often leave a person feeling exhausted, the far infrared sauna is usually quite energizing. Research conducted largely in Japan suggests that the far infrared sauna has a wider range of therapeutic effects than traditional saunas or steam baths, especially for detoxification.

FASTING DETOXIFICATION

Fasting is not for everyone and one should always consult with a physician knowledgeable about fasting before beginning. Fasting is not for expectant mothers, diabetics and others with a history of medical problems. There are other options such as eating programs of cleansing foods or specific balancing diets for metabolic imbalances (we will discuss these in later chapters).

WHAT IS A FAST?

The dictionary definition of a fast is the practicing of abstaining from food, either completely of partially, for a specific period of time. Traditionally fasting has been widely used for the purpose of purifying the person or atoning from misdeeds.

During a fast, a metamorphosis occurs as the body undergoes a tearing down and rebuilding of damaged tissues. There is a remarkable redistribution of nutrients in the fasting body. While it breaks down and eliminates old tissue, toxins and inferior materials, it retains essential vitamins and minerals. The end result is a thorough cleansing of the digestive tract, its membrane and cellular structures. This process of cleansing and rebuilding has made fasting popular for its ability to rejuvenate, heal certain disease and give the body a more youthful appearance.

Eliminations during the cleansing process

- Dead, dying or diseased cells
- Unwanted fatty tissue
- Trans-fatty acids
- Hardened coating of mucus on the intestinal wall
- Toxic waste matter in the lymphatic system and bloodstream

- Toxins in the spleen, liver and kidneys
- Mucus from the lungs and sinuses
- Imbedded toxins in the cellular fibers and deeper organ tissues
- Deposits in the microscopic tubes responsible for nourishing brain cells
- Excess cholesterol

The Result

- Mental clarity is improved
- Rapid, safe weight loss is achieved without flabbiness
- The nervous system is balanced
- Energy level is increased
- Organs are revitalized
- Cellular biochemistry is harmonized
- The skin becomes silky, soft and sensitive
- There is greater ease of movement
- Breathing becomes fuller, freer and deeper
- The digestive system is given a well-deserved rest

There are many different types of fasts which can basically be divided into one of two categories: Normal fast or Partial fast.

- A "normal fast" is going without food for a definite period during which you ingest only liquids (water and/or juice). The duration can be 1 day, 3 days, 1 week, 1 month or 40 days. Extreme care should be taken with fasts lasting longer than 14 days and should only be attempted after medical advice from your physician. Examples of these types fast would be the "lemonade fast" or "juice or vegetable broth fast".

- A "partial fast" is one that omits certain foods or designates a schedule that includes limiting food, such as eating one meal per day or of omitting one meal a day. An example is eating only fresh, "chemical-free" vegetables or cleansing fruit for several days.

During a fast there are several stages of the cleansing process that takes place in the body.

The first stage of cleansing removes large quantities of waste matter and digestive residues. Your bathroom may be your best friend that day and you may also feel headachy, mild nausea and sweaty as the residues of waste matter are released and some passing into the bloodstream.

The second stage is the cleansing of mucus, fat, diseased and dying cells, and the more easily removed toxins. The cleansing process becomes more thorough as each day passes. By the third day of the fast, there is little desire for food, the tongue becomes coated and the breath foul as the body excretes waste through every pore on the body.

The last stage is the cleansing of toxins that have been accumulating in the cells of the body since birth. Cleansing at this stage is only possible through a combination of juice fasting, water fasting in sufficient quantities to flush toxins being released from fat.

To heal from illness, the body redirects all of its resources toward cleansing and repairing by removing appetite and virtually shutting down digestion. This is the reason why there is little desire to eat food when one is sick—the body wants to focus all of its resources on cleansing in order to heal.

There is a mental and spiritual component to fasting especially when the fast extends greater than three days.

There is a definite and obvious mental effect on the brain and senses. When University of Chicago students fasted for seven days, mental alertness increased and their progress in schoolwork was cited as *remarkable*. A universal testimony of fasters is that thinking is enhanced. The mental and physical senses are heightened, and often, there can be a feeling of euphoria, especially during longer fasts. Some will experience more emotional stability because they have eliminated overeating secondary to emotional dependence on food, excluded stimulant foods like caffeine, processed sugars and trans-fatty acids, all of which can have a tumultuous effect on emotions.

Spiritually, fasting is a powerful discipline for bringing the body under submission. Each great servant of God has had his/her time of fasting. It is an essential spiritual discipline and without it we are weak. It fortifies spiritual foundations, builds intimacy with God and strengthens resolve. Fasting with prayer allows us to hear from God and move past our fears and step out on faith into the place where God has called us. If you are spiritually asleep, fasting and prayer will restore that fiery passion in you. If you are seeking direction, truth will be revealed. If you are in a spiritual battle, fasting gives the edge for victory. If you have a request before God, there is no position more powerful than fasting in humility and praise.

IMPORTANT PRECAUTIONS

Again, let me reiterate precautions to fasting;

1. This is something that should be done for a short period (defined as 48 hours) unless you are under the supervision of a health professional who understands the physiology of fasting. Even one and two-day fasts require guidance if you have never attempted one before.
2. Anyone with a serious health problem should NOT fast unsupervised unless they have experience of the process. This includes anyone who is diabetic or pregnant.

3. Anyone who is currently taking prescription medication should not fast unless under the supervision of an expert.

4. Anyone who has a history of eating disorders such as anorexia or bulimia should not fast unless under supervision.

DETOXIFICATION SUPPORT METHODS

There are a number of other supportive measured to assist the detoxification process which have a proven beneficial effect. They include:

- Hydrotherapy
- Salt bath soaks
- Dry brushing
- Lymphatic and therapeutic massage
- Aerobic exercises (rebounder)
- Breathing and relaxation techniques

Heretofore, detoxification programs have been utilized as a healing treatment for various serious illnesses, but ideally it should be the primary tool of prevention. In other words, "Don't wait for the shoe to drop" before you begin to take care of yourself. Establish a routine schedule for cleansing your body the same as you would clean your house, your clothes or your car.

PREVENTION IS THE KEY!

PEARL NUMBER TWO

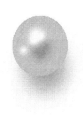

∫∫ IMMUNITY – FOUNDATION FOR PREVENTION ∫∫

The immune system is composed of many interdependent cell types that collectively protect the body from bacterial, parasitic, fungal, viral infections and from the growth of tumor cells. Many of these cell types have specialized functions. The cells of the immune system can engulf bacteria, kill parasites, or kill viral-infected cells, as well as destroy other internal hazards such as cancerous cells, arteriosclerotic plaque, cholesterol deposits and free radicals.

There are two lines of defense:

- Our skin, mucus secretions, and stomach acid act as the first barrier against unwanted germs called **Innate immunity**
- Our body's ability to retain a memory of all the invaders it has faced, which allow the body to be infected only once, even after repeated exposure to the disease called **Adaptive immunity**.

Len Saputo, M.D. states in his book, "Harmful Flora," that if the gastrointestinal tract becomes unbalanced and the liver detoxification system breaks down, our entire immune system can malfunction in three ways:

- A weakened immune system can result in immune suppression diseases, such as cancer and AIDS.
- The overburdened immune system can overreact and become hyperresponsive to normal stimuli; this occurs in asthma, migraine, and food allergies.
- A malfunctioning immune system can cause auto-immune reactions, when antibodies target our own tissues, as in rheumatoid arthritis or lupus.

The gastrointestinal tract is the largest immune organ in our body. 80 percent of all our protective immune globulins are produced in the digestive tract. It isn't difficult to see that when this large, strategically placed immune system member isn't working well, our defenses are lowered. Once our barriers are down, it becomes more difficult to defend against invaders.

One of the reasons medicine does not focus on the immune system is that its parts and interconnectedness are not readily perceivable. We can see and understand the workings of the digestive system, the circulatory system, the nervous system, and the respiratory system. These systems are easily described because they are physically connected. The immune system, on the other hand, consists of apparently unrelated parts and pieces, and much of their connections are cellular.

IMMUNE SYSTEM COMPONENTS

- **Bone Marrow** -- All the cells of the immune system are initially derived from the bone marrow. The bone marrow produces B cells, natural killer cells, granulocytes and immature thymocytes, in addition to red blood cells and platelets.

- **Thymus** -- The function of the thymus is to produce mature T-lymphocytes which are then released into the bloodstream and serve as the first line of defense against tumor cells and infections.

- **Spleen** -- The spleen is an immunologic filter of the blood. It is made up of B cells, T cells, macrophages, dendritic cells, natural killer cells and red blood cells. In addition to capturing foreign materials (antigens) from the blood that passes through the spleen, migratory macrophages and dendritic cells bring antigens to the spleen via the bloodstream for destruction.

- **Lymph Nodes** -- The lymph nodes function as an immunologic filter for the bodily fluid known as lymph. Lymph nodes are found throughout the body and are composed mostly of T cells, B cells, dendritic cells and macrophages. They drain fluid from most every tissue in the body.

CELLS OF THE IMMUNE SYSTEM

- **T-Cells** -- T lymphocytes are usually divided into two major subsets: the T helper cells called the CD4+ T cell and the T killer/suppressor also called the CD8+ T cell. The T helper cells main function is to augment or potentiate immune responses by the secretion of specialized factors that activate other white blood cells to fight off infection. The T killer/suppressor cells are important in directly killing certain tumor cells, viral-infected cells and sometimes parasites. Both types of T cells can be found throughout the body, in the lymph nodes, spleen, liver, lung, blood, and intestinal and reproductive tracts.

- **Natural Killer Cells** -- Natural killer cells, often referred to as NK cells, are similar to the killer T cell. They function as effector cells that directly kill certain tumors such as melanomas, lymphomas and viral-infected cells, most notably herpes and cytomegalovirus-infected cells.

- **B Cells** -- The major function of B lymphocytes is the production of antibodies in response to foreign proteins of bacteria, viruses, and tumor cells. Antibodies are specialized proteins that specifically recognize and bind to one particular protein. Antibody production and binding to a foreign substance or antigen, often is critical as a means of signaling other cells to engulf, kill or remove that substance from the body.

- **Granulocytes or Polymorphonuclear (PMN) Leukocytes** -- Another group of white blood cells is collectively referred to as granulocytes or polymorphonuclear leukocytes (PMNs). These cells are predominantly important in the removal of bacteria and parasites from the body. They engulf these foreign bodies and degrade them using their powerful enzymes.

- **Macrophages** -- Macrophages are important in the regulation of immune responses. They are often referred to as scavengers or antigen-presenting cells (APC) because they pick up and ingest foreign materials and present these antigens to other cells of the immune system such as T cells and B cells. This is one of the important first steps in the initiation of an immune response.

- **Dendritic Cells** -- These cells are usually found in the structural compartment of the thymus, lymph nodes, spleen and also in the bloodstream and other tissues of the body. It is believed that they capture antigen or bring it to the lymphoid organs where an immune response is initiated.

IMMUNE SUPPRESSION

The stepchildren of the immune system are the tonsils and the appendix. They have been poorly understood by the medical community and by routinely removing them may account for the greatest contributor to immune suppression in the body. The tonsils happen to be one of the first lines of defense against disease, and possibly your only defense against the poliomyelitis virus.

Another medical procedure responsible for suppressing the immune system is the appendectomy (removal of the appendix). Appendicitis is actually a warning of something even bigger amiss in the body. Removing inflamed tonsils or an inflamed appendix is equivalent to tossing out your smoke detector because it's making too much noise. Immunologists now tell us that the tonsils are not to be removed under any circumstance, yet even today, there will be over a million tonsillectomies performed in America. In some states, removing the appendix is required by law if the lower abdomen is opened. Fortunately, 20% of the time we actually grow back tonsils and appendices after they've been removed.

Here are some other circumstances that depress immunity:

1) All surgeries depress the immune system. The greatest cause of death following a successful surgery is a secondary, or nosocomial infection (one picked up as a result of the hospital stay). With a depressed immune system, secondary infections are deadly.

2) Antibiotics depress the immune system by taking over its job. Antibiotics also deplete the "good" bacteria (probiotics) needed for cleansing toxins from your system.

3) Corticosteroids have been (and are still) administered abundantly because of their anti-inflammatory properties, although the use of corticosteroids is a double edged sword: they suppress the initial inflammatory response to injury or illness, but they also suppress the immune system.

4) Chemotherapeutic agents, radiation and many pharmaceutical medications are among the greatest suppressors or disablers of immunity.

5) Poor Nutrition

6) Negative stress - For a long time psychologists were aware of the impact stress had on the body's ability to fight infections, but now a study has shown how stress also plays a major influence in altering the functions of the immune system. 293 stress-related studies were performed between the years of 1960 and 2001 with 18,941 subjects being evaluated in the studies.

Findings of studies on immunity vs. stress–

- Periods of short-term stress triggered the immune system to prepare for injury or infection, similar to a "flight or fright" response
- Long-term stress caused excessive wear on the body and activated a deterioration of the immune system
- The immune systems of the elderly and those already suffering with some kind of illness were less capable of coping with stressful situations

Researchers concluded that:

1) The stressors that most negatively compromised the immune system were the chronic stressors.

2) They also discovered the longer the duration of stress or perceived length of the stress, the less the body's ability to adapt to the stressful situation.

It was determined that this kind of negative stress could lead to serious negative health repercussions beginning with attacking the immune system at the cellular level then going after the overall broader functions of the immune system. The immune system is action and reaction. It has an intelligence of its own.

IMMUNITY AND ENERGY FIELDS

Aberrant energies always exert an immunosuppressive influence on the human system by upsetting the delicate balance of internal bioenergies upon which immunity depends. Aberrant energies can invade the human energy system from external sources such as exposure to microwaves, radiation, fluorescent lights and other forms of electromagnetic pollution, or they can be generated internally by emotional turmoil, toxins, ailing organs, or obstructed energy channels.

Energy Factors That Impair Immunity

1) **Abnormal electromagnetic fields** - We have already discussed in detail the hazards to human health generated by power lines, electrical appliances and a growing array of electronic gadgets. By suppressing the pineal and pituitary glands and impeding cerebral functions, abnormal electromagnetic fields impair immunity at its central headquarters in the brain.

2) **Microwaves** - Not only do microwaves suppress the same glands and tissues as abnormal electromagnetic fields, but they also constitute a primary stimulant of the human stress response. Passive exposure to

microwave radiation triggers stress response in even the calmest most balanced individuals. In laboratory tests conducted on rats, exposure to microwaves at levels **twenty times below** the current safety standards set in the USA provoked sufficient stress to exhaust and cause a complete breakdown of their immune system.

3) **Air pollution** - Air pollutants such as motor-vehicle exhaust, smoke and industrial emissions fill the air with heavy positive ions that negate the activity of negative ions, the tiny charged particles which hold atmospheric energy and carry it into the human system via breath.

Air conditioning and central heating have the same effect, robbing the air in closed buildings of vital negative-ion energy. Unless you compensate for such "dead" air with internal energy practices such as an ionizer, your immune system will gradually wind down leaving you chronically fatigued and vulnerable to the mildest pathogens.

4) **Deficient light** - Light is the primary source of energy for the pituitary gland, which receives the energy through the retina and optic nerve. Light also influences the pineal gland and is required by the body to produce vitamin D. Light also regulates many human biorhythms, particularly sleep.

"Full-spectrum light" is the type light that nourishes the body and contains all the wavelengths of natural sunlight. Not only is an ordinary light bulb deficient in many vital frequencies, but the light from fluorescent tubes and television screens vibrate erratically and tend to irritate the pituitary gland and the central nervous system via the optic nerve. Numerous studies conducted in American schools have shown that many of the abnormal behavior patterns and learning impediments which increasingly impair classroom discipline and education in the USA are quickly corrected when fluorescent lights are replaced with full-spectrum lights.

5) **Shallow breathing and physical stagnation** - Lack of sufficient exercise and shallow breathing create conditions of chronic fatigue and physical stagnation in the human body, lowering resistance and impairing immunity. Depriving the body of sufficient oxygen impedes circulation, restricts distribution of nutrients and inhibits cellular metabolism.

6) **Emotional turmoil** - Frequent outbursts of extreme emotions are regarded as the primary internal source of disease in traditional Chinese medicine. Emotional equilibrium is a precondition for maintaining strong immunity and nothing throws human energy off balance more quickly and extremely than sudden outbursts and prolonged bouts of uncontrolled "energies." It is well known that grief such as that experienced after the death of a spouse, renders a person highly vulnerable to disease and degeneration. Fortunately, there are simple and effective ways to remedy and prevent assaults on the immune system in concert with along targeted nutritional support program.

OPTIMIZING IMMUNE FUNCTION

By far, the most important factor in maintaining an effective immune response is controlling your body's pH (acid-alkaline) balance. Normal blood pH works within a very narrow parameter of 7.35 – 7.45 pH, which is critical to health, wellness and life. Our body's cells, organs and systems function most effectively in an alkaline environment and are degraded in an acidic environment. In other words, an acidic tissue pH is destructive and toxic, whereas an alkalinity enhances and rejuvenates the body. Another way to look at it from a diet prospective: an <u>acidic diet</u> is the basic "meat and potatoes," whereas an <u>alkaline diet</u> is a meal of "fruits and vegetables." Fast foods, traditionally cooked foods, processed foods all acidify the body while most fruits and raw or lightly sautéed vegetables alkalinize the body.

UNDERSTANDING ACID-ALKALINE BALANCE

It is very important to have a chemical balance between these acid and alkaline conditions, both in the blood and in the tissues. The acid and alkaline conditions are opposites, and when they are balanced, they cancel each other out. However, it is very easy for the body tissues to become too acidic, and this imbalance sets the stage for disease.

In scientific terms, the acid/alkaline relationship is known as pH. The pH of the body has a profound effect on the inner environment and the microscopic organisms. The pH of blood and tissues is a critical number and ideally should be approximately 7.35. The pH of saliva and urine should be approximately 7.2 or higher. Understand that urine is an excretion product of the tissues not the blood, so when you are testing the pH of the urine you are actually testing the pH of the tissues. Therefore, when your urine pH is over 7.2 then the body tissues are alkaline and healthy. When the pH of the urine is below 7.2 then the body tissues are acidic and unhealthy.

THE BATTLE FOR PH BALANCE

There is a great battle going on inside each of us and we don't even know it! Our body is waging a daily war against bacteria, virus, fungus, yeasts, and molds. As killer bugs and bad bacteria get stronger and stronger, our immune systems are becoming weaker and over-taxed in this war. Even the medical profession's first line of defense (the antibiotic) is becoming less and less effective against new resistant strains created daily as bacteria mutate.

The key to maintaining superiority in this conflict is an uncompromised immune system-digestive tract, lymph system, blood, urinary tract and interstitial fluids. Our bodies are alkaline by design and acid by function. Maintaining proper alkalinity is essential for life, health, and vitality. To put it simply, an imbalance of alkalinity creates a condition favorable to the growth of bacteria, yeast and other unwanted organisms.

Medical biochemists and physiologists have recognized pH (acid-alkaline) balance as the most important aspect of a balanced and healthy body. They have long known that the maintenance of an alkaline pH in our tissues and cells is critical to cellular health. The only exceptions are our digestive tract which has varying degrees of acid by design, (except for our normally alkaline mouth) and our urinary tract which should be slightly acidic for healthy function.

We live and die at the cellular level. All the cells (billions of them) that make up the human body are slightly alkaline, and must maintain alkalinity in order to function and remain healthy and alive. As each alkaline cell performs its task of respiration, it secretes metabolic wastes, and these end products of cellular metabolism are acid in nature. These waste acids must not be allowed to build up; otherwise, sickness and disease are inevitable. It is widely believed that the immune system is the body's first line of defense, but in actuality it is not. Instead, we must look at pH balance as the first and major line of defense against sickness and disease.

ALKALIZE

An Alkaline Diet

Almost all foods that we eat, after being digested, absorbed, and metabolized, release either an acid or an alkaline base into bloodstream. Grains, fish, meat, poultry, shellfish, cheese, milk, and salt all produce acid, so the introduction and dramatic rise of our consumption of such foods meant that the typical Western diet became more acid-producing. The consumption of fresh fruit and vegetables continually decreased, which further contributed to the acidic Western diet.

The theory behind the alkaline diet is that our diet should reflect physiological pH (7.35 to 7.45) which is slightly alkaline. Proponents of alkaline diets believe that a diet high in acid-producing foods disrupts this balance and promotes the loss of essential minerals such as potassium, magnesium, calcium, and sodium, as the body tries to restore equilibrium. This imbalance is thought to make people prone to illness.

Review the charts on the following pages to better understand alkaline foods versus acidic foods. The goal is to balance acidic foods with alkaline foods in an effort to achieve optimal physiological pH.

A SIDE NOTE: This approach to eating is linked to of the practice of food combining; the purpose of food combining is to facilitate digestion--to make it easier, less complicated, and more efficient, possibly avoiding or even eliminating digestive problems. The digestion of different foods requires different arrays of glands, enzymes, juices in the digestive secretions.

ALKALIZING FOODS

VEGETABLES
Garlic
Asparagus
Fermented Veggies
Watercress
Beets
Broccoli
Brussel sprouts
Cabbage
Carrot
Cauliflower
Celery
Chard
Chlorella
Collard Greens
Cucumber
Eggplant
Kale
Kohlrabi
Lettuce
Mushrooms
Mustard Greens
Dulce
Dandelions
Edible Flowers
Onions
Parsnips (high glycemic)
Peas
Peppers
Pumpkin
Rutabaga
Sea Veggies
Spirulina
Sprouts
Squashes
Alfalfa
Barley Grass
Wheat Grass
Wild Greens
Nightshade Veggies

FRUITS
Apple
Apricot
Avocado
Banana (high glycemic)
Cantaloupe
Cherries
Currants
Dates/Figs
Grapes
Grapefruit
Lime
Honeydew Melon
Nectarine
Orange
Lemon
Peach
Pear
Pineapple
All Berries
Tangerine
Tomato
Tropical Fruits
Watermelon

PROTEIN
Eggs
Whey Protein Powder
Cottage Cheese
Chicken Breast
Yogurt
Almonds
Chestnuts
Tofu (fermented)
Flax Seeds
Pumpkin Seeds
Tempeh (fermented)
Squash Seeds
Sunflower Seeds
Millet
Sprouted Seeds

OTHER
Apple Cider Vinegar
Bee Pollen
Lecithin Granules
Probiotic Cultures
Green Juices
Veggies Juices
Fresh Fruit Juice
Organic Milk (unpasteurized)
Mineral Water
Alkaline Antioxidant Water
Green Tea
Herbal Tea
Dandelion Tea
Ginseng Tea
Banchi Tea
Kombucha

SWEETENERS
Stevia

SPICES/SEASONINGS
Cinnamon
Curry
Ginger
Mustard
Chili Pepper
Sea Salt
Miso
Tamari
All Herbs

ORIENTAL VEGETABLES
Maitake, Reishi
Daikon
Dandelion Root
Shitake, Kombu
Nori, Wakame,
Sea Veggies
Umeboshi

ACIDIFYING FOODS

FATS & OILS
Avocado Oil
Canola Oil
Corn Oil
Hemp Seed Oil
Flax Oil
Lard
Olive Oil
Safflower Oil
Sesame Oil
Sunflower Oil

FRUITS
Cranberries

GRAINS
Rice Cakes
Wheat Cakes
Amaranth
Barley
Buckwheat
Corn
Oats (rolled)
Quinoa
Rice (all)
Rye
Spelt
Kamut
Wheat
Hemp Seed Flour

DAIRY
Cheese, Cow
Cheese, Goat
Cheese, Processed
Cheese, Sheep
Milk
Butter

NUTS & BUTTERS
Cashews
Brazil Nuts
Peanuts
Peanut Butter
Pecans
Tahini
Walnuts

ANIMAL PROTEIN
Beef
Carp
Clams
Fish
Lamb
Lobster
Mussels
Oyster
Pork
Rabbit
Salmon
Shrimp
Scallops
Tuna
Turkey
Venison

PASTA (WHITE)
Noodles
Macaroni
Spaghetti

OTHER
Distilled Vinegar
Wheat Germ
Potatoes

DRUGS & CHEMICALS
Chemicals
Drugs, Medicinal
Drugs, Psychedelic
Pesticides
Herbicides

ALCOHOL
Beer
Spirits
Hard Liquor
Wine

BEANS & LEGUMES
Black Beans
Chick Peas
Green Peas
Kidney Beans
Lentils
Lima Beans
Pinto Beans
Red Beans
Soy Beans
Soy Milk
White Beans
Rice Milk
Almond Milk

IONIZED OR ALKALINE WATER

Ionized water is the product of mild electrolysis which takes place in the ionized water unit. Ionized water is treated tap water that has not only been filtered, but has also been reformed in that it provides reduced water with a large mass of electrons that can be donated to active oxygen in the body to block the oxidation of normal cells. To realize the importance of alkaline or ionized water, the most important feature of water produced by a water alkalinizer, Oxidation Reduction Potential (ORP), must be understood. ORP is the electrical potential of a substance expressed in millivolts. This tells us how well that substance is able to donate electrons. Water with a high negative ORP is of particular value in its ability to neutralize oxygen free radicals. Water coming directly from the tap had an ORP of +200 to +400mV, while the water coming out of the water alkalinizer had a negative ORP. The more negative the ORP of a substance (e.g., the higher its negative ORP), the more likely it is to engage in chemical reactions that donate electrons. These electrons are immediately available to engage in reactions that neutralize positively charged free radicals.

Drinking a glass of ionized/alkaline water is like drinking a glass of anti-oxidants. It delivers a massive amount of negatively charged electrons that neutralize the free-radicals causing daily damage & progressive aging within your body (Toxic chemicals, poor diet, stress, air and water pollution, medications, etc. are constantly bombarding us with free radicals). This is the key benefit of water produced by a water alkalinizer.

Ionized water restores alkalinity and flushes acidic toxins from the body, leaving the blood cleaner and better able to transport nutrients to the cells.

Acidic blood is filled with yeasts, molds, bacteria, and the wastes they produce as well as the waste produced by the cells of our body through digestion and metabolism.

Disease cannot thrive in an alkaline environment and although water mixed with bicarbonate is indeed alkaline, it does not have a negative ORP; rather its ORP is positive, meaning it is unable to neutralize dangerous oxygen free radicals.

In the world we live in today, ***everyone is too acidic*** and we all need to alkalize. Nearly every diseases or condition associated with aging such as diabetes, high blood pressure, arthritis, cancer, arthritis, chronic fatigue, even the skin losing elasticity (wrinkling) can develop and accelerate within an acidic body.

Inside a water ionizer, filtered water is passed by electrically charged platinum coated titanium plates. As water passes between the plates, the positive charged ions (cations) are attracted to the negative plate and vice versa. The negative charged ions provides the powerful anti-oxidant effect. The electrolysis process also reduces the cluster size from about 10 to 13 water molecules per cluster down to about 5 to 8 molecules per cluster.

OTHER USES FOR ALKALINE WATER

There are many more benefits to "alkaline water" than simply the alkalinity or pH. In addition, alkaline water has an incredible surfactant/cleaning capability. Alkaline water is also excellent for cooking fish, vegetables, meat, and rice. It brings out the real taste in food because it does not break it down like acid water. Alkaline water eliminates the bitter taste of coffee and tea.

Investing in an alkaline ionizer is a vital purchase that will pay off in preventive health benefits that will be measured by your superior quality of life.

OTHER ALKALIZING TOOLS

Green Drink

A green drink is any leafy green vegetable such as romaine lettuce, kale, spinach, chard or collards blended into two quarts of spring water. Preparing a green drink daily is a simple, but excellent way to alkalize and oxygenate the body.

To make your own "green drink", place a handful of red or green or bib or romaine lettuce leaves (never use ice berg) in the blender with three or four cups of water. Liquefy for about two or three minutes. You can strain it if you like, or keep the fiber in. Put in a squirt of fresh lemon juice if you like, or add Trace Mineral Drops to further increase pH. Put it into a water bottle and sip it throughout the day. Always make a fresh batch daily.

Bicarbonate of Soda

Your body pH can also be boosted by adding a ¼ teaspoon of baking soda (bicarbonate) to your drinking water when your diet or stress creates excessive acidity.

Testing Your pH

The first step in establishing a health-promoting alkaline diet is to assess your current first morning urine pH. This is a good measure of your average body pH and is easily obtained with pH testing strips. pH test strips measures acid-alkaline states ranging at least from 5.5 to 8.0.

First thing in the morning, upon first urination, wet the tape either by urinating directly on the tape or by collecting the urine in a cup and dipping the tape into the urine. Match the color of your test strip with the color chart on the back of the test tape packet. Any number below 7 indicates that your urine is on the acidic side. The lower the number, the more acidic you are. 7.0 indicates the neutral state and 7.4 would be an ideal first morning urine pH.

Other major factors that contribute to an acidic body are stress and acidic drinking water. We will discuss these in more detail in later chapters.

MINERALIZE – FOR OPTIMAL IMMUNE FUNCTION

IODINE – THE UNIVERSAL NUTRIENT

Iodine is referred to as the universal nutrient because it is found in every cell in the body. It is known as the element necessary for thyroid hormone production, but in fact, it is also responsible for the production of all the other hormones in the body. Iodine contains powerful antibacterial, antiparasitic, antiviral and anticancer properties and adequate levels are necessary for healthy immune function. It elevates pH levels and is a mycolytic agent. Iodine has also been effective for treating fibrocystic breast and ovarian cyst.

Other conditions treated with iodine are ADD, atherosclerosis, breast disease, excess mucus production, fatigue, hemorrhoids, headaches (migraine), hypertension, infections, keloids, liver disease, parotid duct stones, prostate disorders, sebaceous cysts and vaginal infections.

Iodine sufficiency was associated with a sense of overall well being, lifting of "brain fog," feeling warmer in cold environments, increased energy, needing less sleep, achieving more in less time, experiencing regular bowel movements and improved skin complexion.

Iodine deficiency disorders result in conditions such as goiter, mental retardation, infertility and increased infant and child mortality. Approximately 1/3 of the world's populations live in iodine deficient areas according to the

World Health Organization. The earth's crust is not very abundant in iodine and the highest percentage is found in seawater, seaweeds and sea organisms. In fact, sea vegetables are among the most concentrated natural sources of iodine.

Experts in the field of inorganic iodine supplementation have established that 12.5 mg iodide/iodine (Iodoral) is sufficient for optimal thyroid and breast health. More may be necessary to address the needs of the rest of the body. Every body is different relative to iodine needs, therefore, an Iodine-Loading Test is recommended to access individual needs and determine daily dosage.

Finally, understand that iodized salt only contains enough iodine to prevent goiter and does not come close to addressing the needs of the entire body. Also, vegan and vegetarian diets, diets that do not include ocean fish or sea vegetables or diets that are high in bakery products (e.g., breads, cakes, pasta, etc.) which contain brominated flour can lead iodine deficiency.

Evaluating and maintaining optimal iodine levels will not only improve immune system function, but also help us achieve optimal health and wellness.

SELENIUM AND ZINC

The minerals selenium and zinc are indispensable to the human immune system, because they are required to manufacture antioxidant enzymes, which protect the body from free-radical damage.

SELENIUM is an essential trace element necessary for regulating thyroid function and iodine metabolism. It is a required component in the function of at least 11 enzymes and without it life would not be possible. One enzyme in particular, glutathione peroxidase, is critical in protecting our body from oxidation damage. Toxic agents such as pesticides, mercury, chlorine and bromine cannot be thoroughly detoxified by glutathione activity in the absence of selenium.

Studies have shown that selenium depletion in individuals result in gastrointestinal disorders such a Crohn's disease. Selenium deficiencies are linked to increased risk of death from lung, colorectal and prostate cancers, arthritis, cardiomyopathy/heart disease and HIV disease progression. It is hypothesized that the potent antioxidant activity of selenium counteracts damage caused by these conditions.

ZINC, an essential mineral found in every cell in the body, stimulates the activity of over 100 enzymes in the body. Some of its many known functions are as follows:

- Detoxifies lead, mercury and cadmium
- Maintains a healthy immune system
- Accelerates wound healing
- Reduces colds
- Maintains sense of taste and smell
- Maintains sight
- Synthesizes DNA
- Supports normal growth and development during pregnancy, childhood, and adolescence,
- Helps sperm develop
- Promotes ovulation and fertilization
- Protects against prostate problems
- Helps protect against cancer
- Helps decrease cholesterol deposits
- Good for hair and skin health
- Helps preserve mental faculties in the elderly

The latest research shows that zinc can also protect us against esophageal cancer. Individuals, who suffer from GERD, in particular, have a higher incidence of developing esophageal cancer and should take at least 15 mg of zinc daily.

Zinc is used to synthesize eighty different enzymes, including the body's most potent anti-aging enzyme, superoxide dismutase.

Other minerals essential for immune function include magnesium, potassium, manganese, sodium, copper and chromium.

MINERAL ASSIMILATION AND pH

Every mineral has its own specific pH level at which it can be assimilated into the body. In other words, pH balance determines the bioavailability of mineral usage by the body. If we look at the periodic table and at the atomic number of elements, those with lower numbers are capable of being assimilated at a broader the pH range than those with higher atomic numbers. Therefore, a mineral such as iodine needs a nearly perfect pH to be assimilated into the body. If body pH is not balanced, i.e. too acidic, then most minerals will simply be rejected. In the case of iodine, this rejection would compromise healthy thyroid gland function. Thyroid dysfunction has been related to arthritis, heart attack, diabetes, cancer, depression, fatigue and obesity.

VITAMINS ESSENTIALS

Vitamins found in the marketplace today exist in two forms: synthetic and a natural form. It is most that you select the correct form and sources.

1. Synthetic vitamins are formed in a laboratory by reconstructing vitamin molecules chemically. They are less expensive and can actually be harmful to your system. Synthetic vitamins can produce drug-like effects and cause the body to try to compensate for missing components.
2. Natural vitamins made from whole foods and food concentrates such as carrot powder, wheat germ, or buckwheat provide nutritional balance. Their molecular and biochemical combinations remain untampered with

and work in partnership with one another as complex nutrients to repair tissues, boost immunity or sustain cell life.

Some manufacturers of vitamin C create it from the synthetic "ascorbic acid" because it's less expensive and lasts longer. Large doses of this material have been found to cause collagen disease, rebound scurvy, kidney stones and impaired mineral metabolism.

The New England Journal of Medicine noted that the smokers in the study who ingested normal doses of "synthetic" vitamin E and beta-carotene actually had a higher incidence of lung cancer, more heart attacks and an 8 percent higher overall death rate.

VITAMINS IMPORTANT TO IMMUNITY

Many vitamins function not only as nutrients, but also as potent antioxidants. When the body is disease-challenged or under severe stress, it utilizes vitamins at a far greater rate than under normal conditions. This fact that shows how important these nutrients are to immune function.

Vitamin C

Vitamin C (ascorbic acid or ascorbate) is nature's most potent antioxidant cofactor. Ascorbate helps to detoxify various drugs and chemicals, is important in wound repair and tissue healing. It helps prevent cancer, counteracts the immunosuppressive effects of cortisone, protects the heart and boosts overall immunity. The optimum maintenance dose is 2-6 grams per day and double that amount when ill.

Here are scientifically shown benefits that ascorbate promotes or enhances:

- Scurvy resistance: improved blood vessel and cardiovascular integrity
- Enhances hormone health and neurotransmitter functions

- Promotes immune system healthy and reduces unhealthy actions
- Enhances and repairs detoxification functions
- Enhances healthy bone formation
- Enhances and rebuilds glutathione functions
- Reduces bioaccumulation of toxins
- Protects DNA from oxidative damage
- Reduces toxic minerals in body
- Enhances natural anti-cancer surveillance

Vitamin D3

Low dietary intake and limited sun exposure have led to an epidemic of vitamin D deficiency. Health experts now advise adults to regularly check their blood levels of vitamin D and to address deficiencies with supplemental vitamin D.

Vitamin D plays many essential roles throughout the body:

- enhancing calcium absorption,
- contributing to healthy bone mass,
- supporting immune function,
- quelling inflammation and
- Helping to fight cancer.

Clinical studies support vitamin D's role in preventing and treating colon and prostate cancers, and emerging studies suggest vitamin D may help avert cancers of the breast, ovaries, head, and neck, among others.

Vitamin D quells inflammation that may exacerbate chronic heart failure, and in combination with other nutrients, benefits people with chronic heart failure.

Vitamin D also shows promise in preventing both type I and type II diabetes, and offers important support for immune health. Vitamin D may help prevent wound infections and flu, support the body's defense against tuberculosis, and boost immune function in patients with kidney failure.

Vitamin D likewise may help to alleviate seasonal affective disorder (SAD), a type of depression experienced during the winter months due to decreased sunlight. Vitamin D appears to be essential in maintaining healthy white blood cells and a robust immune system.

A recent paper presented persuasive evidence that seasonal infections such as influenza may actually be the result of decreased vitamin D levels, not of increased wintertime viral activity, which has been the longstanding conventional wisdom. This makes sense, because vitamin D receptors are present on many of the immune system cells responsible for killing viruses and deadly bacteria, and the vitamin—which is less environmentally available in the winter—appears to be a requirement for proper activation of these cells.

Other immunity-boosting vitamins include, in order of potency, vitamins A (preferably as beta-carotene), vitamin E and vitamin B1, B5, B6, and B12.

AMINO ACIDS

Arginine, when taken with synergistic cofactors such as vitamin B, stimulates the pituitary to secrete growth hormone, a vital immune regulator. Arginine also enlarges the thymus gland (which produced T-cells), greatly enhances the body's healing powers and helps prevent cancer.

Other immune-boosting amino acids include ornithine, cysteine, taurine, methionine and glutathione.

PHYTOCHEMICALS

Phytochemicals are non-essential plant chemicals that have protective or disease preventive properties. There are more than thousand known phytochemicals. It is well-known that plants produce these chemicals to protect themselves, but recent research demonstrates that they can protect humans against diseases as well. Some of the well-known phytochemicals are lycopene in tomatoes, isoflavones in soy and flavanoids in fruits. They are not essential nutrients and are not required by the human body for sustaining life.

Structures of different types of phytochemicals

There are many types of phytochemicals and each type works differently. Listed below are some the some possible actions:

- **Antioxidant** - Most phytochemicals have antioxidant activity and protect our cells against oxidative damage and reduce the risk of developing certain types of cancer. Phytochemicals with antioxidant activity: allyl sulfides (onions, leeks, garlic), carotenoids (fruits, carrots), flavonoids (fruits, vegetables), polyphenols (tea, grapes).
- **Hormonal action** - Isoflavones, found in soy, imitate human estrogens and help to reduce menopausal symptoms and osteoporosis.
- **Stimulation of enzymes** - Indoles, which are found in cabbages, stimulate enzymes that make the estrogen less effective and could reduce the risk for breast cancer. Other phytochemicals, which interfere with enzymes, are protease inhibitors (soy and beans), terpenes (citrus fruits and cherries).

- **Interference with DNA replication** - Saponins found in beans interfere with the replication of cell DNA, thereby preventing the multiplication of cancer cells. Capsaicin, found in hot peppers, protects DNA from carcinogens.
- **Anti-bacterial effect** - The phytochemical allicin from garlic has anti-bacterial properties.
- **Physical action** - Some phytochemicals bind physically to cell walls thereby preventing the adhesion of pathogens to human cell walls. Proanthocyanidins are responsible for the anti-adhesion properties of cranberry. Consumption of cranberries will reduce the risk of urinary tract infections and will improve dental health.

Foods containing phytochemicals are already part of our daily diet. In fact, most foods contain phytochemicals except for some refined foods such as sugar or alcohol. Some foods, such as whole grains, vegetables, beans, fruits and herbs, contain many phytochemicals.

The easiest way to get more phytochemicals is to eat more vegetables such as broccoli, cauliflower, cabbage, Brussels sprouts, and turnips, are rich in beta-carotene and protect mucous membranes, especially in the lungs and intestinal tract, from cancer and free-radical damage. Also fruits such as blueberries, blackberries, cranberries, pomegranate, wolfberries, cherries, apples, acai, wild strawberries, noni and olives have potent immunity-boosting properties when consumed regularly in sufficient quantities. The most recent recommendations are to eat 9 to 13 servings of fruits and vegetable daily.

Garlic is probably the foremost immune-enchanting food one can eat. It has a wider spectrum of antibiotic activity than penicillin, inhibits many viruses and helps prevent cancer. It is also one of the richest natural sources of selenium, which is required to produce the potent antioxidant enzyme gluthione peroxidase. It is most effective when consumed raw.

HERBS

Many herbs have potent immune-boosting properties. The North American herb Echinacea (purple Kansas cornflower) is also a highly effective immune-system tonic and was widely used by the Plains Indians to cure and prevent many ailments. Other North American herbs that boost immunity are chaparral (Larrea divaricata), yerba mansa (Anemopsis californica) and osha (Ligusticum porteri).

The South American herb pau d'arco (Tabebuia pentaphylla) enhances the body's ability to resist pathogens and also directly attacks outside invaders.

In Chinese medicine, the most widely used herbs for enhancing immunity are ginseng, ginkgo, astragalus, gotu kola, ligustrum and codonopsis. Shiitake, maitake, reishi and other Chinese mushrooms also have strong immunity-enhancing properties and are frequently included in herbal formulas that boost immunity.

Cordyceps Sinensis is a fungus that grows in the high altitudes of the Tibet, Nepal and parts of China. Although technically not a mushroom, it has been a staple of Traditional Chinese Medicine (TCM) for over 1500 years, prized by Chinese Nobility for its healing powers, subject of over 300 clinical studies and credited for helping Chinese Olympians shatter track and field records.

Some of the more prominent uses for Cordyceps are increasing energy, endurance and stamina; battling weakness and fatigue; boosting lung function and oxygen capacity; boosting the immune system and improves sexual function

Cordyceps sinensis is an adaptogen herb. An adaptogenic herb **must help build resistance to all areas of stress that may affect our body**. Finally, an adaptogen herb will be able to normalize the body and place the body in proper balance. **The key with an adaptogen is being able to adapt to**

what the body needs and balancing the body.

PROBIOTICS

Probiotic supplements such as acidolphilus, bifidus and fermented cabbage juice replenish the colonies of "friendly" bacteria in the intestinal tract. Lactobacteria are the body's only natural defense against candida and other yeast infections, which have powerful immunosuppressive properties. They also facilitate rapid elimination of toxic digestive wastes and improve assimilation of essential nutrients from food.

SOIL BASED ORGANISMS or SBOs perform the same job in the digestive tract as they do in soil. In the GI tract, SBOs maintain the balance against bad bacteria, which can quickly gain the upper hand. Even the slightest imbalance results in bad gas, or diarrhea. Digestion is a time sensitive process; too fast or too slow causes gastrointestinal stress. Left unattended, chronic GI imbalances like constipation, IBS, and Crohn's Disease can develop.

Dannon launched a heavy advertising campaign suggesting that eating Dannon yogurt would help you live long, healthy life. Unfortunately, there are numerous problems with dairy-based probiotics ranging from lactose intolerance, growth hormones and antibiotics contained in commercial grade milk to a limited shelf life of dairy-based probiotic strains.

SBOs are the best alternative to dairy-based probiotics and were virtually unknown until about 9 years ago. Although still a well-kept secret to the average consumer, it is indisputable that SBOs are the superior probiotic. **They are essential to restore and maintain optimum GI health** and daily administration **increases mental and physical performance** plays a major role when dealing with **immune diseases,** as well as the **toxic effects of chemotherapy and cancer medications**, whose side effects include severely diminished bowel function.

PEARL NUMBER THREE

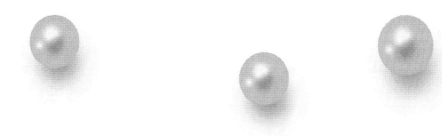

ʃʃ THE NEW-TRITION PROBLEM ʃʃ

PROCESSED FOODS – THE "NEW" FOOD

Let's stop here just for a moment to access the nature of the sustenance we call food. It is clear that the manna we eat usually originates from a natural source, but when we process it, we actually alter its quality, nutritional value and character. What we end up with biologically is a "new food," i.e., a deviation of what was created in nature. Any modification in the biochemistry of foods modifies its effect and value to the body and therefore its purpose in the body. We know that "natural food" theoretically has not been manipulated in any way and the term "processed" in today's language is applied to assure us that somehow the food has been made better. In the early era of modern agribusiness (the mass production of food) "processed" meant simply cleaning and washing of produce or the packaging food in its "raw" state. Over time food became less connected to agriculture and more associated with business, which determined that profit was the goal and no longer high quality nutritious sustenance. The turning point was when science was applied to the agricultural industry. This was not a bad thing when it was applied for the correct purpose, i.e., to support the production of the highest quality nutritious produce. Unfortunately, in a very short period of time, food science was directed toward maximizing production and retarding spoilage with minimal concern about nutrition.

Today, when we see processed foods, it rarely resembles the source from which it came and more significantly has only minuscule nutrition value to the body. Be sure to understand that food in its "original" form is all about nutrition to the body and all else is secondary. The "new food" is absolutely about business profit in the form of addictive taste (high sugar vs. high salt), strategic marketing (appealing packaging, target groups) and convenience to the consumers without regard to health considerations. What kind of sophisticated marketing campaigns have you seen to get us to buy carrots, kale, walnuts or cold water fish? Again, it goes back to the fact that the "new foods" are developed to be income vehicles to their manufacturers.

FAST FOOD FACTS

Courtesy of **SUPER SIZE ME**

- Each day, 1 in 4 Americans visits a fast food restaurant
- In 1972, we spent 3 billion a year on fast food - today we spend more than $110 billion
- Most nutritionists recommend not eating fast food more than once a month
- French fries are the most eaten vegetable in America
- You would have to walk for seven hours straight to burn off a Super Sized Coke, fries and Big Mac
- Eating fast food may be dangerous to your health

RESULTS OF A FAST FOOD DIET

- Former Surgeon General David Satcher: "Fast food is a major contributor to the obesity epidemic"
- 60 percent of all Americans are either overweight or obese
- The World Health Organization has declared obesity a global epidemic
- Left unabated, obesity will surpass smoking as the leading cause of preventable death in America
- Obesity has been linked to: Hypertension, Coronary Heart Disease, Adult Onset Diabetes, Stroke, Gall Bladder Disease, Osteoarthritis, Sleep Apnea, Respiratory Problems, Endometrial, Breast, Prostate and Colon Cancers, Dyslipidemia, steatohepatitis, insulin resistance, breathlessness, Asthma, Hyperuricemia, reproductive hormone abnormalities, polycystic ovarian syndrome, impaired fertility and lower back pain
- One in every three children born in the year 2000 will develop diabetes in their lifetime
- Diabetes will cut 17-27 years off your life

As you can easily see, obesity and diabetes are the two main symptoms of a chronic fast food diet and are the doorway to a host of disorders and diseases.

FOOD SECURITY

DEFINITION - Food security exists when all people, at all times, have physical and economic access to sufficient, safe and nutritious food to meet their dietary needs and food preferences for an active and healthy life.

Food security includes the ready availability of nutritionally adequate and safe foods. The keyword in our society today is "safe." Safety in our food supply can only be accomplished when we know the "chain of custody" from the seed to the table. Unfortunately, most of us have no idea of how are where our food came from or what happened to it along the way.

Here is an excerpt written by Charlie Jackson called," *Taking Back Control of Our Food Sources"* that sums up the definition of food security and it importance to every human being.

What's happening to our food? How did it happen that cows are routinely fed chicken litter, hormones and antibiotics, and parts of other cows? Why does our food travel an average 1,500 miles and many days from the farm to the dinner table while local farmers are going out of business? Why are pigs and chickens raised in cages so small that they can barely turn around and have to have their tails cut off or their beaks clipped in order to keep down the stressed induced mutilations? Why do we have outbreaks of hepatitis from imported green onions? And why is there massive destruction and loss of soils, heavy chemical and fuel inputs, and an agriculture system based on industrial models? Why is there an epidemic of obesity and diabetes, particularly among people who can least afford food? Why are foods genetically engineered but not labeled as such? Labels are something that over 90% of Americans want on their prepared foods. And why are we losing our farmers, losing them so rapidly that there are now more people in the United States in prison than there are farming the land? The answer is that we have lost control of our food system.

For the last 10,000 years or so, all of agriculture was local. Most of our grandparents grew up eating food that they grew themselves, or they knew the farmer that grew the food. Only in the last couple of generations has there been such a radical disconnect from the food that we eat and the farmers that produce it. This has led to a massive concentration in food production, with food becoming just another global commodity, and the near total loss of control on the part of the consumer. Most food production is now out of sight and thus out of mind. That's why good people of good conscience end up supporting a system that is bad for farmers, bad for farm animals, bad for the land, and bad for the consumers.

And our tax dollars support this massive concentration of farms and the system that makes the foods that are the least healthy for us the cheapest. It is a bitter irony that most of the subsidies to agriculture, subsidies that come from our tax dollars, go to farmers growing corn for corn sugar and grains for meat. This means that almost all prepared foods--from soda to pasta sauce--now contain corn sweetener. It also means that grain-fed meat--meat very high in fat--is extremely cheap. Americans are consuming massive amounts of these prepared foods and cheap fatty meats and getting more overweight and unhealthy. At the same time we are experiencing an epidemic of obesity, an epidemic that is already consuming everyone's dollars through increased health costs, and now tax dollars are being used directly to address this epidemic.

We can take back our food system. The one sure way to make certain you are not supporting the current destructive industrial agriculture system is to buy locally grown food. Getting to know the person who grows your food is a powerful way to reconnect with food and community--when you support your local farm, you get the freshest food, keep money in the local economy, and make sure that we keep farms as part of our landscape, while making sure that you have a say in how the food is grown.

But they're still not fresh. They've also most likely lost 50 percent of their nutritional value by the time they hit your plate. And regardless of what the folks in the ad department tell you, they *don't* taste like

Grandma's tomatoes.

It has been postulated that food should travel from the field to your kitchen in the same amount of time it takes to travel through your digestive system. That can't happen when the lettuce in your salad comes from Salinas, Calif.

Studies show that most of the food we eat travels about 1,200 miles before it gets to our mouths.

Whenever I meet someone from another country, I ask about the kind of food they eat at home and where their fresh produce comes from. What I find amazing is that, six times out of 10, they know that their food comes from a local source. Even more incredibly, these foreigners often know the name of the farm or farmer who produces the food they eat. These are not necessarily agriculturally attuned individuals; they seem to know (or know of) the folks who grow their food the same way that I know the guy who works on my truck, or the woman at the local convenience store where I buy my morning coffee on the way to work.

In America, I doubt whether more than one person in 5,000 knows the farmer who grows the veggies or meat they consume. Here, knowing where your fresh groceries are grown is akin to knowing where the coffee you get from a machine at a rest area along the interstate comes from. There doesn't seem to be much sense of responsibility on the part of whoever produces that vending-machine coffee – and you can tell by the taste. By the same token, there isn't much incentive to produce good-tasting veggies when the person who ends up eating them is some faceless nonentity living halfway across the country.

FOOD ADDITIVES... SUBTRACT!

The primary dangers with processed and fast foods are hydrogenated oils used to extend the shelf life of foods and high fructose corn syrup(HFCS) for its addictive qualities.

Food additives are another "red flag" of potential hazards to your health as many are already found on the CDC's list of known carcinogens.

Question:

> Would you go to a restaurant or diner, blindfold yourself (since you cannot see food additives), nose clip your nose (you cannot smell additives) and eat from a menu of foods with names you need Chemistry 102 to pronounce?

> Would you take medicines from prescription pill bottles with names written in unknown languages?

This is exactly what happens when we eat processed foods trusting that the ingredients inside are safe because the packaging outside is pretty, colorful and appealing. The manufacturer uses marketing misnomers like "natural," "healthy," "heart healthy," "enriched," "whole wheat," "high fiber," "zero calories" just to name a few, when these terms are all relative because there are no set standards or basis for these terms. How "high" is high fiber when it is compared to the minimum daily allowance for dietary fiber? What is enriched flour "enriched" with and why does it have lower nutrient value than unprocessed flour? Is it deceptive to use the term "whole wheat" when it does not refer to "100% whole wheat"? A prime example of potentially misleading inference is "contains zero calories." The only naturally-occurring (God-made) substance in nature with zero calories is "water." Putting anything else labeled "zero calories" into our bodies would be "UNCIVILIZED" or definitely unnatural. All marketing terms for food packaging are approved or sanctioned by the FDA, but curiously does not carry the same definition as we may assume. Many additives are considered "safe" by our government can be found on the Center for Disease Control and Prevention (CDC) list of carcinogenic agents.

The only sure way to avoid potentially harmful additives in your diet is to read the label of virtually every processed food you buy. A rule of thumb is… if a food label has more than three ingredients beware. If more than five, know each ingredient, otherwise, avoid it altogether.

Here is a list of a <u>few</u> food additives that will give you some idea of the inherent dangers of additives in our food:

A. ARTIFICIAL FLAVORINGS

Coumarin--Used for 75 years in imitation vanilla before it was found to produce liver damage in animals.

Piperonal--An inexpensive substitute for costly vanilla flavoring. It is used industrially to kill lice.

Butyraldehyde--Used for a nutty flavor. Industrially, it is an ingredient in rubber cement and synthetic resins.

Aldehyde C-17--Used for a cherry taste. It is a flammable liquid used industrially in aniline dyes, plastics, and synthetic rubbers.

Ethyl Acetate--Used for a pineapple flavor. The vapor can cause chronic lung, liver, and heart damage. This chemical is used industrially as a solvent for plastics and lacquers.

Mesityl Oxide--Used for color and flavor. This is a petroleum-based compound found in lubricating oils, insecticides, plastic wrapping material, can linings, adhesives, inks, and varnishes. It has the characteristic odor of the urine of tomcats and is sometimes detected in some of the plastic food wrapping material you might have around the house.

Monosodium Glutamate (MSG)--Early in this century a Japanese chemist identified MSG as the substance in certain seasonings that added to the flavor of protein-containing foods. Unfortunately, too much MSG can lead to headaches, tightness in the chest, and a burning sensation in the forearms and the back of the neck. Also, avoid <u>hydrolyzed vegetable protein</u>, or HVP, which may contain MSG.

B. ARTIFICIAL COLORING

The definition of artificial coloring is any non-food substances added to food to change its color. The American food industry uses 3000 tons of food color per year.

People learn to associate certain colors with certain flavors, and this causes the color of food to influence the perceived flavor, in everything from fruit gum to wine. For this reason, food manufacturers add dyes to their products. While most consumers are aware that foods with bright, unnatural colors, like Froot Loops, are artificially colored, few people know that apparently "natural" foods such as oranges are sometimes also dyed to mask natural variations in color.

In the United States, certifiable color additives are available for use in food as either **"dyes"** or **"lakes."**

Dyes dissolve in water, but are not soluble in oil. Dyes are manufactured as powders, granules, liquids or other special purpose forms. They can be used in beverages, dry mixes, baked goods, confections, dairy products, pet foods and a variety of other products.

Lakes are the combination of dyes and insoluble material. Lakes tint by dispersion. Lakes are not oil soluble, but are oil dispersible. Lakes are more stable than dyes and are ideal for coloring products containing fats and oils or items lacking sufficient moisture to dissolve dyes. Typical uses include coated tablets, cake and donut mixes, hard candies and chewing gums.

Artificial dyes and preservatives are widely used in foods, beverages, and drugs. The most common coloring agents are azo dyes: tartrazine (orange), sunset yellow, amaranth and the new coccine (both red); and the non-azo dye pate blue.

Red Dye No. 2 (Amaranth)--One of the many coal tar dyes; but Amaranth has gained universal acceptance. Principal uses have been in beverages, but it is also widely used in candy, confections, pet food, dessert powders, bakery goods, sausages, ice cream, sherbet, dairy products, cereals, snack foods, etc. Allergists have reported cases of Amaranth sensitivity. The Russians have done extensive research on this synthetic food coloring and have found that it not only tends to produce cancer, but could cause malformed and softened fetuses (unborn babies). It was finally banned in 1976; however, it is supposed to be replaced by Red Dye No. 40, which is as bad or worse than Red Dye No. 2.

See Appendix I for a comprehensive list of current, widely used food colorings.

OTHER FOOD COLORING ADDITIVES

Alginic Acid--Used in cheese spreads to give uniformity of color and flavor. It is used industrially in making artificial ivory and celluloid.

Beta-Naphthylamine--This is used to make two coal-tar dyes to color butter and oleomargarine. Has caused bladder cancer in animals.

Disodium EDTA--Used to promote color, flavor, and texture retention in canned carbonated soft drinks, distilled alcoholic beverages, vinegar, canned white potatoes, clams, crabmeat, and shrimp. Also in cooked canned mushrooms, various canned beans, pickled cucumbers and cabbage, and in liquid multi-vitamin preparations. It is also used in beer, mayonnaise, margarine, potato salad, and sandwich spreads, etc. In the human body, it inhibits enzymes and blood coagulation, causes gastrointestinal disturbances, muscle cramps, and kidney damage.

C. ARTIFICIAL SWEETNERS

Aspartame (NutraSweet, Equal)--Accounts for more than 75% of all adverse reactions reported to the FDA's Adverse Reaction Monitoring System (ARMS). Many reactions to aspartame were very serious including seizures and death. Other adverse reactions reported included:

- **Headaches/Migraines, Dizziness, Weight gain, Memory loss, Muscle spasms, Joint Pain, Nausea, Numbness, Depression, Fatigue, Irritability, Tachycardia, Heart palpitation, Insomnia, Vision Loss, Hearing Loss, Breathing difficulties, Tinnitus, Vertigo, Anxiety attacks, Slurred Speech, Rashes, Loss of taste.**

The following list contains a selection of chronic illnesses, which may be triggered or worsened by ingesting of aspartame (Mission Possible 1994)*:

- **Brain tumors, Multiple sclerosis, Epilepsy, Chronic fatigue syndrome, Parkinson's disease, Alzheimer's, Mental retardation, Lymphoma, Birth defects, Fibromyalgia, Diabetes.**

H.J. Roberts, MD, coined the term "aspartame disease" in a book filled with over 1,000 pages of information about the negative health consequences of ingesting aspartame.

Latest Update:

New Italian Study Confirms: Aspartame is a Carcinogen

June 19 2007

A new study of the Cesare Maltoni Cancer Research Center of the European Ramazzini Foundation has not only confirmed but further reinforced the results of an earlier study by the same research institute that found the artificial sweetener Aspartame to cause cancers and leukemia in rats. The earlier study was condescendingly dismissed by industry and by the European Food Safety Agency as well as US FDA, but evidence of the damage done by the sweetener does not seem to be going away. If anything, the scientific findings overwhelmingly suggest that there are real problems that can no longer be brushed under the carpet.

Dr. Morando Soffritti's research was conducted for 36 months using 1,800 rats. It forced the conclusion that aspartame is a multipotential carcinogen. Cancers aspartame produced included leukemia, lymphoma, kidney, and cranial peripheral nerves among others. Only the rats fed aspartame got malignant brain tumors. This prodigious work was peer reviewed by 7 world experts.

This work confirmed studies presented to the FDA 25 years ago that documented a catalogue of brain, uterine, ovarian, testicular, mammary, pancreatic and thyroid tumors. Based on the evidence FDA **denied approval of aspartame** for 16 years from the time it was discovered.

Splenda™-- The artificial sweetener sucralose, which is sold under the name Splenda™, is one of the up-and-coming "next generation" of high-intensity sugar substitutes. Sucralose is produced by chlorinating sugar (sucrose). A lot of the controversy surrounding sucralose stems from the fact that it was discovered while trying to create a new insecticide. The claim that it is made from sugar is a misconception about the final product.

One small study of diabetic patients using the sweetener showed a statistically significant increase in glycosylated hemoglobin (HbA1C), which according to the FDA implies a lessening of control of diabetes.

Research in animals has shown that sucralose can cause many problems in rats, mice, and rabbits, such as:

> **Shrunken thymus glands (up to 40% shrinkage), Enlarged liver and kidneys, Atrophy of lymph follicles in the spleen and thymus, Increased cecal weight, Decreased red blood cell count, Hyperplasia of the pelvis, Extension of the pregnancy period, Aborted pregnancy, Decreased fetal body weights and placental weights, Reduced growth rate, Diarrhea.**

According to the book *Sweet Deception*...

> Sucralose is made when sugar is treated with trityl chloride, acetic anhydride, hydrogen chlorine, thionyl chloride, and methanol in the presence of dimethylformamide, 4-methylmorpholine, toluene, methyl

isobutyl ketone, acetic acid, benzyltriethlyammonium chloride, and sodium methoxide, making it unlike anything found in nature. The Splenda website even states that "although sucralose has a structure like sugar and a sugar-like taste, it is not natural." The product Splenda is also not actually calorie-free. Sucralose does have calories, but because it is 600 times sweeter than sugar, very small amounts are needed to achieve the desired sweetness.

The name sucralose is another misleading factor. The suffix *-ose* is used to name sugars, not additives. Sucralose sounds very close to sucrose, table sugar, and can be confusing for consumers. A more accurate name for the structure of sucralose was proposed. The name would have been trichlorogalactosucrose, but the FDA did not believe that it was necessary to use this so sucralose was allowed. Sucralose is not yet approved for use in most European countries, where it is still under review.

Sweet and Low--Several studies in the 1970s linked saccharin with cancer in laboratory animals. Avoid it. Sweetener packets and cans of saccharin-containing diet drinks bear warning labels: *"Use of this product may be hazardous to your health. This product contains saccharin, which has been determined to cause cancer in laboratory animals."* Saccharin sold as "Sweet and Low" was found to be directly linked to bladder cancer in laboratory animals.

Acesulfame K--Known commercially as Sunette or Sweet One, acesulfame is a sugar substitute sold in packet or tablet form, in chewing gum, dry mixes for beverages, instant coffee and tea, gelatin desserts, puddings and non-dairy creamers. Acesulfame K does contain the carcinogen methylene chloride. Long-term exposure to methylene chloride can cause **headaches,**

depression, nausea, mental confusion, liver effects, kidney effects, visual disturbances, and cancer in humans. There has been a great deal of opposition to the use of acesulfame K without further testing, but at this time, the FDA has not required that these tests be done.

D. PRESERVATIVES

The most commonly used preservatives in food are sodium benzoate, 4-hydroxybenzoate esters, and sulfur dioxide. Various sulfites are commonly used in prepared foods. It is estimated that 2-3 mg of sulfites are consumed each day by the average U.S. citizen, while an additional 5-10 mg are ingested by wine and beer drinkers. The largest sources are salads, vegetables (particularly potatoes), and avocado dip served in restaurants.

Sodium Benzoate--A deadly poison used as a preservative in soda pop, jams, jellies, pickles, and countless other so-called foods. Sodium Benzoate kills or inhibits all living organisms present within the jar or other container. We are living organisms too, but because of the small doses in food products, the harmful effects may not become evident until years later.

Sodium Nitrate and Sodium Nitrite-- Used as a preservative and color fixative in cured meats, meat products, and certain cured fish, such as bacon, bologna, hot dogs, deviled ham, meat spreads, potted meats, almost all ham, sausages, smoked and cured shad, salmon, tuna fish products, poultry, wild game, pickled corned beef, tongue, pastrami, and a host of cold cuts. Meats, no matter in what stage of decay, are kept a pinkish color, which implies freshness. If most of the meats did not have these two chemicals within, most people would probably not buy the product, since it would resemble a gray, colorless cadaver (corpse). The danger is that sodium nitrite tends to lessen the blood's ability to carry oxygen and if ingested in sufficient quantities can lead to respiratory failure.

Butylated Hydroxyanisole (BHA) and Butylated Hydroxytoluene (BHT) These are two of the most widely used antioxidants in foods, which stabilize fats so they don't become rancid due to their loss of natural antioxidants in factory processing. BHA is in almost every processed food that the "average person" eats.

BHT is used in as many foods as BHA. For example: cereals, rice, shortenings, potato flakes, sugar, cured meats, potato chips, etc. These two chemicals are also used in making plastic packaging material, rubber gaskets, milk cartons, wax paper, and lubricants. Both have caused dermatitis (skin disease), severe allergic reactions such as disabling chronic asthmatic attacks, skin blistering, eye hemorrhaging, tingling of face and hands, extreme weakness and fatigue, edema (swelling), chest tightness, and difficulty in breathing.

Acetic Acid -- Used as a dip for shrimp and other fish meats to prevent discoloration. It is also used in the manufacturing of plastics and dyeing of silks.

Sulfites--Sulfites are a class of chemicals that can keep cut fruits and vegetables looking fresh. They also prevent discoloration in apricots, raisins, and other dried fruits; control "black spot" in freshly caught shrimp; and prevent discoloration, bacterial growth, and fermentation in wine. Until the early 80's they were considered safe, but CSPI found six scientific studies proving that sulfites could provoke sometimes severe allergic reactions. CSPI and the Food and Drug Administration (FDA) identified at least a dozen fatalities linked to sulfites. All of the deaths occurred among asthmatics. In 1985 Congress finally forced FDA to ban sulfites from most fruits and vegetables. Especially if you have asthma, be sure to consider whether your attacks might be related to sulfites. The ban does not cover fresh-cut potatoes, dried fruits, and wine.

Calcium or Sodium Propionate--Retards molding and spoilage in breads; it is a fungicide.

Coal-Tar Derivative Paraffin--Coats fresh fruits and vegetables to prevent spoilage.

E. STABILIZERS

Propylene Glycol--A stabilizer used in ice cream, candies, synthetic whipped toppings and in almost everything processed that the "average person" eats. This chemical is used in germicides, paint removers and antifreeze substances.

Sodium Carboxymethylcellulose--Used as a cheese stabilizer and as a thickener in ice cream and whipped topping mixes. It is found in resin emulsion paints and, printing inks. It can cause intestinal obstruction and has produced arterial lesions (diseases in the arteries) similar to high blood cholesterol.

Potassium Bromate--This additive has long been used to increase the volume of bread and to produce bread with a fine crumb (the non-crust part of bread) structure. Most bromate rapidly breaks down to form innocuous bromide. However, bromate itself causes cancer in animals. The tiny amounts of bromate that may remain in bread pose a small risk to consumers. Bromate has been banned virtually worldwide except in Japan and the United States. It is rarely used in California because a cancer warning might be required on the label.

F. OILS

Partially Hydrogenated Oil--Prevents rancidity and deterioration in commercial peanut butters and scores of processed foods and candies. It alters the biological qualities in food. In this case, the vegetable oil is subjected to an extremely high temperature and in the presence of a metal catalyst such as nickel or platinum; hydrogen gas is bubbled through the oil, causing its saturation or hardening. The result is a smelly, axle grease-like mess that has to be bleached, filtered, and deodorized. All of the essential fatty acids in the original oil are destroyed.

Unlike butter, hydrogenated oils contain high levels of **trans fats**. A trans fat is an otherwise normal fatty acid that has been changed by the high-heat processing of a "free" oil. The fatty acids can be double-linked, cross-linked, bond-shifted, twisted, or messed up in a variety of other ways. In short, trans fats are poisons, just like arsenic or cyanide. They interfere with the metabolic processes of life.

Brominated Vegetable Oils--Used in soft drinks for uniform distribution of fruity flavors. This has shown evidence of inducing damage in the liver, heart, thyroid, and kidneys of rats and interferes with normal fat metabolism.

G. OTHER ADDITIVES

Caffeine--Found naturally in tea, coffee, and cocoa. It is also added to many soft drinks. It is one of the few drugs -- a stimulant -- added to foods. Caffeine promotes stomach-acid secretion (possibly increasing the symptoms of peptic ulcers), temporarily raises blood pressure, and dilates some blood vessels while constricting others. Excessive caffeine intake results in "caffeinism," with symptoms ranging from nervousness to insomnia. These problems also affect children who drink between 2 to 7 cans of soda a day. Caffeine may also interfere with reproduction and affect developing fetuses. Experiments on lab animals link caffeine to birth defects such as cleft palates, missing fingers and toes, and skull malformations.

Caffeine is mildly addictive, which is why some people experience headaches when they stop drinking it. While small amounts of caffeine don't pose a problem for everyone, avoid it if you are trying to become or are pregnant. And try to keep caffeine out of your child's diet.

The bottom line on most food additives is that they are petroleum-based chemical products and the human body is biologic in by design. The common sense correlation of using chemicals food additives in the food we eat would be to use maple syrup (sugar) as an additive to the gasoline we put into our automobile. It would definitely cause problems in the automobile and eventually complete failure, although the gasoline may have a more appealing "earth-tone" appearance and a pleasant "mapley" fragrance when filling up at the pump.

ABSOLUTELY NO TO GMO

(GENETICALLY MODIFIED ORGANISMS)

Approximately ten years ago, Americans began eating genetically engineered food. Don't be surprised because no one told us. While other countries require mandatory labeling of these food ingredients, our FDA has decided we don't need to know.

Genetic Engineering (GE) is a radical new technology that manipulates the genes and DNA - the building blocks of all living things. Unlike traditional breeding, genetic engineering creates new life forms that would never occur in nature, creating new and unpredictable health and environmental risks. To create GE crops, genes from bacteria, viruses, plants, animals and even humans have been inserted into plants like soybeans, corn, canola, and cotton.

Multinational chemical companies like Monsanto have taken our staple crops and altered them in order to patent and profit from them by increasing their chemical and seed sales and gaining control over farmers and the food chain

107

itself. The same companies that brought us DDT, PCBs and Agent Orange now expect us to trust them with our food supply.

Genetic engineering involves crossing species which **could not cross in nature**. For example, genes from a fish have been inserted into strawberries and tomatoes.

RISKY BUSINESS FOR THE BODY

When a producer or manufacturer of a GE product says there is no evidence that it may be harmful, don't be the first in your neighborhood to use the product.

Consider these factors:

1) Monsanto's Roundup Ready soybeans are herbicide-tolerant plants engineered to survive Roundup weed killer, but what about the health of consumers who eat genetically modified beans?
2) A study published by the Journal of Nutrition in March 1996 showed that there is a significant difference in fat, carbohydrates, ash and some fatty acids of GE soybeans as compared to conventional soybeans.
3) Other findings raised questions about allergens. Allergic reactions are most commonly triggered by undigested proteins. The danger to many humans who are allergic to certain foods is assured, because no one will know what they are eating. For example, for a person deathly allergic to peanuts, a GMO may have a gene from a peanut in it. The allergic person could have a reaction from eating anything that contained the peanut gene.

Here are other examples of GE technology…

Veggie with rat gene

A rat gene has been introduced in broccolini to enhance vitamin C levels. Broccolini is a cross between broccoli and a Chinese kale, and took eight years to develop. The new plants contain up to seven times the quantity of vitamin C, and it is thought that similar experiments would probably be successful with other plants such as rice and tomatoes. Broccolini retains color and stays fresh longer and could eventually help overcome vitamin deficiencies. [Trends in Plant Science 2000, 5:189, Vol. 5, No. 5, May 2000]

Terminator Chicken

A US biotech company plans to create a strain of chicken genetically engineered to have an extra large breast to yield more meat, with a DNA copyright tag inserted among its genes to stop anyone breeding it without permission.

If successful, the firm, AviGenics, based on the campus of the University of Georgia in Athens, would be one of the first to enable GM meat to appear on US supermarket shelves, opening up new tensions with Europe over genetic engineering in food.

To keep proprietorial control over these valuable new animals, AviGenics is working on a novel kind of trademark, a unique sequence of DNA which would be introduced into the chicken's genes. The "trademark" would not only be locked into each of the chicken's millions of cells, but would be handed on to the bird's offspring indefinitely. [GUARDIAN (London) Monday July 31, 2000]

TOXIC EFFECTS OF GENETICALLY ENGINEERED FOODS

One genetically engineered soy developed by Pioneer Hybrid was found to be allergenic and could have killed people with life-threatening allergies if it wasn't, by chance, caught and kept off the market. Since GE soy came on the market, soy allergies have risen 50%. In 1989, 37 people died and thousands were permanently damaged after ingesting a genetically engineered food supplement, GE tryptophan. Beneficial insects, such as monarch butterflies and ladybugs, have also died after eating GE crops.

Even for the 30% of GE products studied for toxicity, the tests were quite limited. For instance, potatoes and corn were engineered to contain a toxin to kill insect pests. These foods are already on the market though no one knows the long-term effects on animals or on humans who eat the "toxin enriched" crops.

TEN USEFUL TIPS TO AVOID GENETICALLY MODIFIED FOODS

While demand for organic food has soared recently, the vast majority of the public are consuming GM-affected foods every day, mainly in the form of GM derivatives and enzymes – which are a potential health risk according to independent geneticists*.

The following tips should help those wishing to <u>avoid</u> GM foods:

1. **READ THE PRODUCT LABEL**S and avoid soy-based ingredients such as soy flour, soybean oil, vegetable oil, lecithin and hydrolyzed vegetable protein. And avoid corn-based ingredients such as modified starch, corn flour, corn starch, corn oil and polenta. Note: These ingredients are to be avoided simply because there is no way of

110

knowing if they contain GM-soy or GM-corn derivatives (unless of course a particular product is guaranteed free of al GM ingredients and derivatives).

2. **BUY YOUR FOOD FROM A RELIABLE SOURCE**: Certified organic products are far less likely to be affected by GM. Look for chemical-free/pesticide-free, locally grown produce from farmers markets and food co-ops.

3. **CUT DOWN ON PROCESSED FOODS** because they are more likely to be affected by GM. In addition, many brands of dairy products, cereals, jam, fruit juice, cooking oil, sweeteners, slimming foods, beverages, wine and beer etc. are produced with GM-enzymes. If you have any doubts about a particular product, contact the manufacturer for assurance – or just leave it out.

4. **AVOID "FAST FOOD" RESTAURANTS** and "low budget" products because GM-foods are being introduced into cheaper brands initially. Home-made meals are obviously far healthier and more nutritious than factory-made equivalents.

5. **BAKERY PRODUCTS** When buying bakery products such as bread, avoid "flour improver" and "flour treatment agent", which may be a mixture of GM-enzymes and additives. The GM enzyme Alpha Amylase is sometimes listed on bakery product labels and is best avoided. Likewise, "ascorbic acid" may be GM-derived. Look for yeast-free organic breads.

6. **DAIRY PRODUCTS** and meat from animals fed GM soy and corn is not labeled as such – in spite of evidence that modified DNA can cross the gut wall and enter spleen, liver and white blood cells. Only use organic milk, butter, cream and cottage cheese etc.

7. **CHOCOLATE** can contain GM-soy lecithin, and "vegetable fat" and "whey" which are affected by GM. Many brands of dried fruit, including raisins, sultanas, currants, dates – and even dried fruit in some breakfast cereals – can be coated with oil derived from GM soy.

8. **SHOP WITH CARE** when buying products such as baby foods, breakfast cereals, soft drinks and slimming foods, as these may well contain added vitamins etc produced from GM-organisms.

9. **REGARDING HEALTH FOOD SUPPLEMENTS**, vitamins and medicines: check with the manufacturer, as some ingredients may be produced by biotechnology. In the USA, the GM food supplement Tryptophan killed 37 consumers and permanently disabled 1,500 more. In addition, for the last ten years there have been reports of a GM version of human insulin causing problems in diabetics who happily used animal insulin for years. (Note: virtually all Vitamin C comes from GE corn)

10. **IS IT REALLY GM-FREE?** When contacting a manufacturer to enquire if a particular product is GM-free, ask them to confirm that the product contains "no genetically modified ingredients or derivatives, and that no GM-derived enzymes were used in its production". Ask for written confirmation rather than relying on verbal assurances.

For more detailed information about the GMO industry read "Seeds of Deception" by Jeffrey Smith.

PHTHALATES - INVISIBLE ENEMY

Phthalates are a class of widely used industrial compounds known technically as dialkyl or alkyl aryl esters of 1, 2-benzenedicarboxylic acid. There are as many uses for phthalates as there are toxicological properties. Phthalates crept into widespread use over the last several decades because of their many beneficial chemical properties.

Intentional uses of phthalates include softeners of plastics, oily substances in perfumes, additives to hairsprays, lubricants and wood finishers. That new car smell, which becomes especially pungent after the car has been sitting in the sun for a few hours, is partly the pungent odor of phthalates volatilizing from a hot plastic dashboard.

Phthalates are ubiquitous, not just in the products in which they are intentionally used, but also as contaminants in every other area of the environment. In fact, we eat so many plastics each day that the government has established an average daily amount that we ingest. Once inside our bodies, these phthalates or plastics tightly hook onto our cell parts where they gum up the works. For example, they damage hormone receptors, leading to loss of sex drive and energy, or they damage brain chemistry leading to learning disability and hyperactivity, or they accumulate in organs and trigger cancers of the prostate, breast, lung and thyroid.

Phthalates and other environmental chemicals are triggers for cancer, but because they resemble our hormone to hormone cell receptors, they gum up the works in ways that are just beginning to understand. **It is no coincidence that the two hormonally linked cancers, breast and prostate, are on a rapid rise and that thyroid medication is the third most commonly prescribed medication in the United States.**

Two phthalates, DEHP and DINP, are of particular concern because they are known to be toxic and sensitive populations could potentially be exposed to them. For instance, premature infants in intensive care units may be exposed to DEHP in plastic medical tubing and bags.

In 2002, the U.S. Food and Drug Administration (FDA) advised that, if available, alternatives to phthalates should be used to keep plastics soft because certain devices could expose people to a toxic dose of DEHP.

The chemical might be found in IV bags and tubing, blood bags, nasogastric tubes, dialysis bags and tubing, and other tubing used to support and feed premature infants, according to the FDA.

In 1999, the European Union banned the use of phthalates from some products, such as baby toys. In the United States and Canada the chemicals have been removed from infant bottle nipples and other products intended to go in a baby's mouth, however the U.S. government has declined to ban the use of phthalates.

THE HEALTH THREAT OF TEFLON CHEMICALS

Teflon, a waxy, white powder, has become a staple in household kitchens everywhere, but this nonstick coating may actually do more harm than good. Accidentally invented by a DuPont chemist more than 65 years ago, Teflon has been raising some health concerns, because of the chemical, perfluorooctanoic acid (PFOA), used to produce it. PFOA has been appearing in people and animals worldwide sited by one study showed that in 23 states, 96 percent of the 598 children tested had traces of the chemical in their blood.

Many studies have been conducted using animals, such as rats, to help answer the question: "Is PFOA a risk to human health?" The studies raised concerns regarding:

- Children's health and development
- Risks of liver, pancreatic, testicular and mammary gland tumors
- Altered thyroid hormone regulation
- Damage to the immune system
- Reproductive problems and birth defects

The research goal is to discover if there is a link between PFOA, hormone levels and liver function.

PFOA has many sources of origin we may not consciously realize such as:

- Teflon manufacturing plants polluting the water and air
- Heating Teflon cookware to broiling temperatures and releasing the chemical into the air
- Vacuuming stain-resistant carpets and emitting chemical infected dust into the air
- Washing stain- or water-resistant clothing, sending chemical coatings down the drain and into the environment

DuPont has been criticized on many sides for its decision not to release all the information it compiled on **perfluorooctanoic acid (PFOA)**. The concerns that:

- **DuPont concealed its own 1981 research showing traces of the chemical in a pregnant worker's unborn child**
- **Ten years later, the company failed to report evidence that the chemical had contaminated the water supply of 12,000 people**

Another health issue, **"Teflon flu"** <u>causes aches and pains when non-stick pans are overheated</u>, although DuPont said the physical problems are temporary and pass quickly. Yet <u>birds, particularly small ones like finches and cockatiels, can die in short order from those kitchen fumes.</u>

DANGERS OF PLASTICS - Trading "Safety" For "Convenience?"

A family of chemicals known as plasticizers is first on the list of potential troublemakers. Plasticizers are used to soften normally hard plastic known as PVC, or polyvinyl chloride. In dozens of animal studies conducted over the past several years, showed that these plasticizers are especially harmful to pregnant mice and their babies. Studies have linked exposure to even low doses of one of these plasticizers, bisphenol-A (BPA), to chromosomal abnormalities. Exposure to the chemical, which creates hormonal imbalances, resulted in everything from high rates of spontaneous abortions to decreased sperm counts in male mice and early onset of puberty in females.

While scientists cannot make the simple leap from mice to men, common sense should definitely raise the red flags of concerns about the potential harm to humans.

Not only do millions of pounds of plastic find their way into landfills every year, 14 percent of air pollution nationwide is from plastic production.

DEPLASTICIZING YOUR FOOD

Chemicals are most likely to migrate from plastic into food when exposed to high heat, harsh soaps, and fat. These precautionary measures can help you play it safe.

1. AVOID MICROWAVING IN PLASTIC

Heat speeds the release of chemicals into food. "People are being sold microwave-safe plastic, when in fact we're not being told what's in there and the rate at which these chemicals leach out," says researcher Frederick von Saal. Avoid this uncertainty by using ceramic or glass instead.

2. EXPLORE THE ALTERNATIVES.

"I have one word for you: glass," says Terry Hassold, a professor of genetics at Case Western Reserve University in Cleveland, who has studied the health effects of bisphenol-A (BPA) on mice. You can also store your food in ceramic containers, waxed- and brown paper bags, and metal canisters made for hot and cold food.

3. USE PAPER--NOT CLING--WRAP.

Many studies indicate that most of the cling wrap used by delis and grocery stores contains high levels of polyvinyl chloride (PVC), a plasticizing chemical that has been linked to hormonal abnormalities in mice. (Happily, the cling wraps made for home use are safer.) Ask the butcher to wrap meat and fish in paper. And transfer fatty deli foods out of plastic wrap and into waxed paper when you get home. "If you put cling wrap that's been plasticized on fatty foods, that stuff will migrate," says Consumer Union's Ned Groth. You might also want to cut off cheese's outer layer-- which has been directly exposed to plastic--before rewrapping it in something safer.

4. WHEN IN DOUBT, THROW IT OUT.

Discoloration, cracks, or other signs of wear suggest your plastic containers are degrading and may be leaching chemicals into your food. Once you've purged your kitchen of old plastic food bins and cups, splurge on a replacement set made of glass.

5. LIMIT YOUR EXPOSURE.

The longer food sits in plastic, the greater its time of exposure to chemicals that could migrate into it. If you must buy food in plastic (and it's hard not to) transfer it into a more food-friendly container (paper or glass) once you get home.

6. WASH PLASTIC BY HAND.

"It only takes 20 washings in the dishwasher for BPA to start leaching," says von Saal. Along with high heat, harsh detergents break down plastic as well. Wash your plastic containers, even those labeled "dishwasher safe," by hand in warm water and mild detergent.

7. READ THE LABEL.

While you'll never find an actual list of ingredients, many plastics come with labels of sorts: those triangles with numbers inside found on the bottom of plastic containers. The numbers you most want to avoid are 3, 6, and 7. The safest numbers are 1, 2, and 5--the type of plastics used in most small water bottles and all soda bottles, yogurt containers, tubs of butter, and so on. (For more details, see "Plastic by the Numbers," page 74.) At the very least, look for brands billing themselves as "PVC-free."

8. BUY GLASS BOTTLES.

Some of the clear plastics, like baby bottles, are treated with bisphenol-A, to which infants are particularly vulnerable. "Using these bottles is like putting a serious drug into what the baby's drinking," says von Saal. Look for glass baby bottles by Evenflo. And avoid drinking water from those five-gallon water jugs delivered to offices and homes, which also contain BPA. Opt instead for filtered water from the tap.

9. BUY IN BULK.

Health food stores are selling everything from pasta to tofu in bulk, and the plastic used to bag bulk products isn't known to be toxic, says Groth. To play it really safe, you can transfer your bagged items to glass containers at home.

PLASTIC BY THE NUMBERS

Many plastics are classified by one of seven codes located in that familiar triangle on the bottom of containers and bottles. (The triangle doesn't mean a plastic container is recyclable; the number inside it simply indicates the kind of resin used.) With plastic wraps and bags, it's harder to know which chemicals have been used. At the very least, look for brands that advertise on their packaging that they don't contain PVC. Until consumers demand better labeling on plastic products, you'll never know exactly what you're getting in your bottles, bins, and bags, but here are a few suspects to try to steer clear of.

#3 Vinyl or PVC (polyvinyl chloride)

Where it lurks: Most commercial cling wrap used in grocery stores and delis; bottles used to store many brands of olive and cooking oils; some water bottles.
Risks: Contains plasticizers that are suspected endocrine disrupters and carcinogens.

#6 PS (polystyrene)

Where it lurks: Some disposable plastic cups and bowls; most opaque plastic cutlery.

Risks: Contains p-nonylphenol and styrene, both of which are carcinogens and suspected hormone disrupters.

#7 "Other" (Usually polycarbonate, or PC)

Where it lurks: Most clear plastic baby bottles, five-gallon water jugs; clear plastic sippy cups; some clear plastic cutlery.

Risks: "Other" is a catchall category, meaning you don't know what you're getting. Most worrisome, many plastics labeled "7" contain bisphenol-A (BPA), an endocrine disrupter.

See Appendix II get a list of stores to purchase safe alternatives to plastics.

H2O, H2O EVERYWHERE,   BUT...

WHICH ONE TO DRINK?

WATER

Water is vitally important to all living things. In the human body water is up to 65 -70 percent water, the brain is composed of 70 percent water, and the lungs are nearly 90 percent water. About 83 percent of our blood is water, which helps digest our food, transport waste, and control body temperature. Every day our body must replace 2.4 liters of water, some through drinking and the rest taken by the body from the foods eaten. Water plays a part in our body's ability to transport these materials all through ourselves. The carbohydrates and proteins that our bodies use as food are metabolized and transported by water in the bloodstream. No less important is the ability of water to transport waste material out of our bodies.

WATER POLLUTION

The majority of the contaminants found in our drinking water can be traced back to excessive or improper use of:

- Gasoline
- Lawn chemicals and
- Prescription drugs.

In short, everything that goes down the drain, onto our lawns or fields or into the air eventually ends up in our drinking water. Most municipal water filtration systems are outdated, (many of them installed in the early decades of the last century) and were not designed to effectively remove these synthetic chemicals. Pesticides and herbicides show up in our tap water now with frightening frequency as well as other chemicals, such as chlorine, chloramine, aluminum, arsenic, and fluoride.

This is the evidence that we must take responsibility for monitoring the safety of our own, personal water supply. Harmful levels of dangerous contaminants simply cannot be detected by sight, taste or smell. Trace levels of some toxins are so dangerous that they are measured in parts per billion and are detectible only by sophisticated laboratory equipment.

Mercury, MTBE, PCBs, Atrazine and Vinyl Chloride are just a few of many the cancer-causing Volatile Organic Compounds (called VOCs) that are found in our water sources nationwide. A fall 2003 study conducted by the State of New Jersey found that 25 percent of the private wells they had tested were contaminated.

In the early 1900s, before the advent of chlorine, pesticides and other chemicals, the average person had a one in 50 chance of getting cancer. Today, one in three can expect to get cancer in their lifetime. The risks are even greater for children. Their systems are still developing and they are getting greater doses of toxins because of their larger consumption of fluids per pound of body weight. They can't detoxify as well as adults, which makes them especially vulnerable.

WATER CHLORINATION

Chlorination of drinking water, combined with the use of sand water filters resulted in the virtual elimination of such waterborne diseases as cholera, typhoid, dysentery and effectively eliminated the outbreak and spread of waterborne diseases.

Chlorine has now been a major part of municipal water treatment for nearly 100 years and approximately 98% of municipal water treatment facilities now use chlorine disinfectant as their disinfectant of choice.

Chlorine is a highly irritating gas destructive to the mucous membranes of the respiratory passages. It is very poisonous & excessive inhalation may cause death. Chlorine is an active bleaching agent & germicide. Both of these effects are due to its oxidizing powers. It is used extensively in the disinfecting of water supplies & in treatment of sewage. American Public Health Association unanimously adopted resolution #9304 in 1993 urging American Industries to discontinuing using Chlorine and virtually all chlorinated organic compounds (e.g. herbicides, pesticides, Splenda, household cleaning products, PVC plastics) because of the serious toxic effects.

Dioxin - An unwanted & undesirable contaminant widely used in herbicides & preservatives is also created by the disposal of synthetic chlorinated organic compounds. The EPA determined in 1994 that the major source of Dioxin contamination in the environment was "medical waste disposal" and urged all health care facilities to explore the ways to reduce or eliminate their use of PVC plastics. Exposure to Dioxin can produce chloracne, liver injury, peripheral neuropathy, central nervous system changes, & psychiatric difficulty. It is carcinogenic in animals at low concentrations. It is one of the most toxic substances to workers exposed in the industrial & agricultural environment. The 1990 Clean Air Act lists Chlorine as a hazardous air pollutant. The EPA has further stated that Chlorine is 300,000 times more potent that the carcinogen DDT which was banned in the US in 1972.

Scientists are now beginning to examine the possible byproducts and side effects of using chlorine in drinking water. Chlorine is listed as a known poison and therefore almost assuredly has an adverse effect on the body. Chlorinated water has been linked to the aggravation and cause of respiratory diseases like asthma and because chlorine vaporizes at a much faster rate than water, chlorinated water presents a significant threat to the respiratory system when used for showering.

Recent discoveries of the health concerns of chlorine have led many people to install shower filters or whole house water filter systems into their homes. Such installations are the next step in the evolution of water filtration technology.

WATER FLUORIDATION

Fluoride may be found in drinking water as a natural contaminant or as an additive intended to provide public health protection from dental caries (artificial water fluoridation). EPA's drinking water standards are restrictions on the amount of naturally occurring fluoride allowed in public water systems, and are not recommendations about the practice of water fluoridation. Since 1945, fluoride has been added to many public drinking-water supplies as a public-health practice to control dental caries.

The practice of fluoridating water supplies has been the subject of controversy since it began (see reviews by Nesin 1956; Wollan 1968; McClure 1970; Marier 1977; Hileman 1988). Opponents have questioned the motivation for and the safety of the practice; some object to it because it is viewed as being imposed on us by the states and as an infringement on their freedom of choice (Hileman 1988; Cross and Carton 2003). Others claim that fluoride causes various adverse health effects and question whether the dental benefits outweigh the risks (Colquhoun 1997).

George L. Waldbutt (founder of allergy clinics in Detroit) did double blind studies with general symptoms noted: Muscle weakness, chronic fatigue, increased thirst, headaches, rashes, joint pain, digestive problems, tingling in extremities, decreased mental acuity.

124

- US National Toxicology in 1989 noted 17% rise in 16 years of Osteosarcoma with males less than 20 years old in fluoridated areas.
- A study done in 84 areas in the US with 39,207 school age children ages 5 - 17 years old with no difference in tooth decay.

When water fluoridation first began it was believed that fluoride had to be ingested for it to be effective. However, this has since changed and the dental community now almost unanimously believes that fluoride's benefits result from topical application, not when it is swallowed.

The fluoride that we ingest from the water supply and from a number of other sources such as toothpaste, mouthwashes, processed food, some vitamin tablets, and beverages like fruit juice, soda and tea is associated with a number of negative health effects. Consider these facts:

- Fluoride accumulates in the bones, making them brittle and more easily fractured, and in the pineal gland, which may inhibit the production of the hormone melatonin, which helps regulate the onset of puberty
- Fluoride damages tooth enamel (known as dental fluorosis) and may lower fertility rates
- Fluoride has been found to increase the uptake of aluminum into the brain and lead into blood
- Fluoride inhibits antibodies from forming in the blood
- Fluoride confuses the immune system, causing it to attack the body's tissues. This can increase the growth rate of tumors in people prone to cancer

Noting these and other health risks and the obvious ethical issue of medicating an entire population without their consent, many European countries have banned water fluoridation.

Austrian researchers further proved in the 1970s that as little as 1 PPM fluoride concentration can disrupt DNA repair enzymes by 50%. When DNA cannot repair damaged cells, we age rapidly. Fluoride prematurely ages the body, mainly by distortion of enzyme shape. Again, when enzymes get twisted out of shape, they cannot do their functions. This results in collagen breakdown, eczema, tissue damage, skin wrinkling, genetic damage, and immune suppression. Practically any disease you can name may then be caused.

We now understand that cancer begins with one cell whose inner blueprint (its DNA) has been disrupted. Without the body's ability to repair its own DNA, a most basic cell function, cancer is promoted, and tumor growth is accelerated.

All systems of the body are dependent upon enzymes. When fluoride changes the enzymes, this can damage:

- immune system
- digestive system
- respiratory system
- blood circulation
- kidney function
- liver function
- brain function
- thyroid function

The distorted enzymes are proteins, but now they have become foreign protein, which we know is the exact cause of autoimmune diseases, such as lupus, arthritis, asthma, and arteriosclerosis.

PHARMACEUTICALS IN OUR WATER

An Associated Press investigation has shown a vast array of pharmaceuticals — including antibiotics, anti-convulsants, mood stabilizers and sex hormones in the drinking water supplies of at least 41 million Americans.

Although the concentrations of these pharmaceuticals are small, (parts per billion or trillion), water utilities insist their water is safe. But the presence of so many prescription drugs and over-the-counter medicines like acetaminophen and ibuprofen in our drinking water has increased worries among scientists over the long-term health consequences.

In the course of a five-month inquiry, the AP discovered that drugs have been detected in the drinking water supplies of 24 major metropolitan areas — from Southern California to Northern New Jersey, from Detroit to Louisville, Ky. Members of the AP National Investigative Team reviewed hundreds of scientific reports, analyzed federal drinking water databases, visited environmental study sites and treatment plants and interviewed more than 230 officials, academics and scientists. They also surveyed the nation's 50 largest cities and a dozen other major water providers, as well as smaller community water providers in all 50 states.

Here are some of the key test results obtained by the AP:

- Officials in Philadelphia said testing there discovered 56 pharmaceuticals or byproducts in treated drinking water, including medicines for pain, infection, high cholesterol, asthma, epilepsy, mental illness and heart problems. Sixty-three pharmaceuticals or byproducts were found in the city's watersheds.
- Anti-epileptic and anti-anxiety medications were detected in a portion of the treated drinking water for 18.5 million people in Southern California.

- Researchers at the U.S. Geological Survey analyzed a Passaic Valley Water Commission drinking water treatment plant, which serves 850,000 people in Northern New Jersey, and found a metabolized angina medicine and the mood-stabilizing carbamazepine in drinking water.
- A sex hormone was detected in San Francisco's drinking water.
- The drinking water for Washington, D.C., and surrounding areas tested positive for six pharmaceuticals.
- Three medications, including an antibiotic, were found in drinking water supplied to Tucson, Ariz.

The situation is undoubtedly worse than suggested by the positive test results in the major population centers documented by the AP.

The federal government does not require any testing or has set safety limits for drugs in water. Of the 62 major water providers contacted, the drinking water for only 28 was tested. Among cities not tested yet were Houston, Chicago, Miami, Baltimore, Phoenix, Boston and New York City's Department of Environmental Protection.

Of the 28 major metropolitan areas where tests were performed on drinking water supplies, only Albuquerque, New Mexico, Austin, Texas and Virginia Beach, Virginia. tested negative.

Even users of bottled water and home filtration systems don't necessarily avoid exposure. Bottlers, some of which simply repackage tap water, do not typically treat or test for pharmaceuticals, according to the industry's main trade group. The same goes for the makers of home filtration systems.

WHAT WATER SHOULD YOU DRINK?

TAP VS. BOTTLED WATER

Tap or Municipal Water (water piped right into your home) must meet the standards of the Environmental Protection Agency (EPA). While the FDA has no authority over tap water, its purity and quality is in the hands of state and/or local authorities.

Water is treated not just to remove disease-causing organisms but also to remove silt, grit and humus material (suspended solids), which can have a detrimental effect upon pipes, meters and other components of the water distribution system. Treating raw water also improves the taste and eliminates objectionable odors or color

Bottled Water is regulated by the FDA which is responsible for the food and pharmaceutical industries. Bottled water is one of the most extensively regulated packaged-food products and receives government oversight from federal and state agencies.

All bottled water types are sometimes referred to as "spring water" but that's not really accurate. The origin and processing of different types of bottled water actually make them quite different in content and taste. In fact, the U.S. Food and Drug Administration (FDA)-the federal agency that regulates all types of bottled water-has established guidelines called standards of identity that classify bottled water into several different water types:

Spring Water is defined as *bottled water derived from an underground formation from which water flows naturally to the surface of the earth.* To qualify as spring water, it must be collected only at the spring or through a borehole tapping the underground formation feeding the spring.

Purified Water is a type of drinking water that has been treated with processes such as distillation, deionization or reverse osmosis. Basically, this means that the bacteria and dissolved solids have been removed from the water by some process, making it "purified." This type of bottled water is usually labeled as *purified drinking water* but can also be labeled for the specific process used to produce it, for example, reverse osmosis drinking water or distilled drinking water. Many bottled water brands are actually purified drinking water.

Mineral Water contains not less than 250 parts per million total dissolved solids and is defined by its *constant level and relative proportions of mineral and trace elements at the point of emergence from the source.* No minerals can be added.

Sparkling Bottled Water contains the same amount of carbon dioxide that it had when it emerged from its source. Sparkling bottled waters may be labeled as *sparkling drinking water, sparkling mineral water, sparkling spring water,* etc.

WATER FILTRATION (especially for municipal water sources)

Reverse osmosis is the best water filtration method known and removes 90-99% of all contaminants (including pharmaceuticals) from city and well water. This process will allow the removal of particles as small as ions from a solution. It is used to purify water and remove salts and other impurities in order to improve the color, taste or properties of the fluid. R.O. technology uses a process known as crossflow to allow the R.O. membrane to continually clean itself, thereby allowing its element to last many years before clogging or needing replacement.

The disadvantage of R.O. water purification is that it removes everything from water, the bad (contaminants) and the good (minerals). Ideally, minerals and trace minerals should be added to replenish the natural chemistry of water making it equivalent to spring water.

THE NEW-TRITION SOLUTION

The convenience of fast foods and prepared foods has robbed us not only of quality family fellowship, but also of our nutritional health and wellness. Ever since Colonel Sanders put the first 12 pieces of chicken in a bucket for us to take home, home food preparation began a slow and sure death. Each time we visit a drive-thru restaurant or eat a frozen TV dinner we are giving control of our health to others not directly concerned about our health.

As individuals and as a society, we are what we eat. Our community landscapes of "golden arches, kings, queens and jacks" are a reflection of our individual and collective diets. The family farm has been replaced by a multitude of fast-food establishments, chain restaurants and big lot grocery stores that rely on food production and distribution systems of industrialized factory farms and large food corporations. Every menu and purchasing decision made by the major fast-food chains shape us and our food system policies even more than the current federal and state farm policies. Like air and water quality, food quality is a critical factor in our personal health and well being.

Each time there is a bacterial contamination scare, only then does anyone critically examine the health quality of our food and food production, processing, and distribution systems.

Convenience and quickness has superseded the primary purpose for which we eat: nutrition and optimal health. It is imperative that we get back to the "garden", eating a wholesome, live, plant-based diet. By making informed lifestyle decisions, i.e., what we will eat and how we will live, we are taking authority of our health and ultimately our life.

WHAT'S IN YOUR BODY?

The most important decision we make each day of our life is not what job or career we pursue in life or even how we manage our finances, but simply what we pick up with our hands and put into our mouths. This daily choice is the key to our quality and quantity of life. In prior generations, this decision process was not as critical because most all foods we ate were natural, fresh and wholesome, free of chemical and manipulations.

In this day and age we are called to stewardship over our own selves. The definition of stewardship simply means we are the responsible party when it comes to our health and wellness. It is a frail excuse to only blame agribusiness or misleading advertisements for our own lack of knowledge and understanding concerning our diet, our nutrition and our food safety. The ultimate responsibility is ours, not our doctor or any other health care professional.

Being a good steward means planning, preparation and the execution of a victorious lifestyle; this begins by making intelligent dietary choices. This approach is optimal health is by your design and is called PREVENTIVE WELLNESS.

Here are five essential points in consideration of "preventive wellness":

READ BEFORE YOU EAT

All packaged, processed foods are required to have labeling so that we can have some idea of what we are consuming. Although in many instances, we still cannot be absolutely sure of what are because of the shrewd marketing and labeling tactics manufacturers employ.

For example, MSG or monosodium glutamate used as a flavor enhancer in foods was found to be responsible for several hypersensitivity reactions based upon an extensive scientific review in 1992 by an independent group of scientists contracted by the Food and Drug Administration (FDA). Their report revealed that MSG-intolerant people with asthma; drowsiness; and weakness experienced symptoms such as burning sensation in the back of the neck, forearms, and chest; numbness in the back of the neck, radiating to the arms and back; tingling, warmth and weakness in the face, temples, upper back, neck and arms; facial pressure or tightness; chest pain; headache; nausea; rapid heartbeat and bronchospasm (difficulty breathing). About 10 years ago, CBS news program, "60 Minutes", broadcast a report exploring hypersensitivity to monosodium glutamate (MSG) and many food producers began using the labeling "No MSG" or "No Added MSG". But careful review of the ingredient label revealed the ingredient hydrolyzed protein, which is also a form of free glutamate as is MSG although significantly less than in amount. Hydrolyzed proteins can be used in a product as leavening agents, stabilizers, thickeners, a protein source, and as a flavor enhancer. When used as a flavoring agent, hydrolyzed proteins are used in the same manner as MSG in many foods such as in canned vegetables, soups, and processed meats. The FDA considers food labeled "No MSG" that contains hydrolyzed protein to be misleading to the consumer. The bottom line is that anyone who is sensitive to MSG or ingredients that contain significant levels of free glutamate should read ingredient labels carefully to screen for ingredients that may cause adverse reactions.

Aside from the potential errors with nutrition labels, product ingredients can also be misleading in other ways. For instance, food products that say they contain milk, fruit or vegetables may not contain them at all. An example is Pillsbury Blueberry Muffins, which do not contain blueberries--they contain artificial blueberry bits.

In addition, allergenic ingredients may not be listed on food labels. Cross contaminations can occur when the same equipment is used to manufacture multiple products potentially causing allergic products to be mixed with non-allergic products.

If the label has words you cannot pronounce…beware! If there are more than three ingredients…be careful; if more than five… beware!

WHAT DID YOU EAT?

So many people we speak to when questioned about their eating habits say things such as, "I eat healthy" or "I eat pretty good". What most people do not realize is that if they eat food from the local grocery or restaurant chain, chances are great that they are unknowingly ingesting hundreds of synthetic substances and toxic chemicals daily. Healthy eating is more than just eating a balanced meal of vegetables, meats and carbohydrates. ***Healthy eating is the practice of making choices about what or how much we eat with the intention of improving or maintaining good health.*** This means following specific guidelines and conscious decisions regarding what you put on your plate and put in your mouth. The decisions to be addressed are:

- increased consumption of foods designated as beneficial;
- decreased consumption of foods designated as detrimental;
- methods of food preparation (e.g., raw versus cooked).
- increased consumption of specific vitamins or other micronutrients
- avoidance of certain food additives (dyes, preservatives, sweeteners);
- avoidance of environmental food contaminants (e.g., mercury, pesticides, herbicides, aflatoxins)
- balance of major nutrients (e.g., proteins, fats, carbohydrates);
- total calorie consumption

Our ideas of what counts as "healthy" is much different from what it was as recent as 10 years ago. The food supply has become a product of the manufacturer's economic decisions rather than our personal health considerations.

Attempting to decipher exactly what certain ingredients are in the foods we eat is another task, but very important. For instance, if you were trying to avoid corn you would have to avoid not only anything listed as corn, but also:

Fructose and fructose syrup	**Malt**	**Baking powder**
Malt extract and syrup	**Sorbitol**	**Maltodextrin**
Monosodium glutamate	**Dextrin**	**Food starch**
Confectioner's sugar	**Starch**	

All of these items could potentially be made from corn, but unless you are specifically aware of what to look for it would be easy to overlook these items when looking for corn on an ingredient label.

EAT TO LIVE vs. LIVE TO EAT

Living to eat can be a form of gluttony. The simplest definition of gluttony is "excessive eating and drinking," but unfortunately there's more to it.

According to Maria Simonson, Ph.D., Sc.D., and director of the health, weight and stress clinic at Johns Hopkins Medical Institutions in Baltimore, stress makes you eat more quickly than anything else. And the foods you want to eat while under stress are more likely to be fatty, pleasurable things that are soft or creamy (aka comfort foods). Hunger is usually not the component of this type of eating.

Excessive eating equals excessive weight gain, which leads to lower self-esteem, higher levels of depression and more stress. It becomes a vicious cycle.

Eating to live means eating under non-stressful circumstances, i.e., not while driving or in transit, or watching the evening news.

Stress stimulated food cravings aren't physiological in nature, but stem from emotional responses (chemical reactions in the <u>brain</u>), and they will continue to torment you until you give in. In fact, these cravings can change as quickly as the emotions that drive them.

EAT 80% RAW

When you eat an abundance of raw fruits and vegetables, they will act as a broom that gently sweeps and cleans the intestinal wall. The colon will be kept squeaky clean. This is important because a clean intestine is necessary for health and to heal disease.

All the nutrients we need can be found in fruits and vegetables. Eating a diet high in raw fruits and vegetables increases energy, assists healing, rebuilds healthy tissue, rejuvenates and invigorates the entire body. You feel vital because all cell functions are operating at peak performance.

Cooking destroys nutrients. Folic acid is abundant in most green vegetables, however, 95% of this vitamin can be lost by cooking. Over 50 fruits and vegetables have oxalic acid. While harmless in its natural state, altered by heat, it becomes harmful. Calcium binds with the oxalic acid in the blood to neutralize it and to form calcium compounds (calcium oxalate) which are difficult for the body to remove and may lead to kidney stones.

Raw food is alkalizing while cooked food is acid-forming. Cooked food tends to have a stimulant effect by causing the body to speed up its metabolism to rid itself of these destroyed nutrients, altered proteins and fats. For anyone going through a health challenge, eating cooked food is like asking runner who just finished a marathon to run 26 more miles uphill in army boots.

WHY RAW?

Although cooking is the traditional method of preparing food, it does not increase nutritional value, but reduces it and actually robs us of vitality. Cooked food causes an increase of white blood cells. The body reacts to cooked food in the same way it reacts to infection. Cooking destroys vitamins, makes minerals inorganic, coagulates proteins, transforms fatty acids, and destroys natural fiber, increasing the transit time through the intestine. This, in turn, causes putrefaction that creates additional toxins.

Research has shown that cooked fiber passes through the digestive system more slowly than raw food. It partially rots, ferments and putrefies, causing toxins, gas and even heartburn. Cooked food is harder to digest, less absorbent, and what is absorbed is not easily assimilated. In short, the body works more for less.

Live Food

Enzymes start to die at 105 degrees, but all are destroyed at 130 degrees Fahrenheit. Food heated over 200 degrees has had nearly all of its phytochemicals denatured or destroyed rendering it lifeless. This is reason leading health authorities agreed that 80% of our diet should be composed of living foods that have not been heated.

We eat living plant foods to consume the enzymes that are a part of the plant's life process. It was once thought that plant enzymes were destroyed in digestion, but these same enzymes can be found in the liver, spleen, heart, lungs, duodenum and urine. When we eat fruits or vegetables, plant enzymes act as catalysts and work in harmony with vitamins, minerals, proteins and fats to nourish every cell of the body. Eating live foods packed with enzymes has a beneficial effect that can be seen throughout the body. Eating a diet high in raw fruits and vegetables increases energy, assists healing, rebuilds healthy tissue, rejuvenates and invigorates the entire body making it operate at peak performance.

When we eat an abundance of raw fruits and vegetables, they act as a broom that gently sweeps and cleans the intestinal wall. The colon is kept squeaky clean which is extremely important for maintaining optimal health and the ability to heal from disease.

DON'T FORGET THE ENZYMES

The power in live food is in the enzymes they carry. Enzymes are vital to life, working tirelessly to break down food and assisting the immune system in carrying out the functions of metabolism. Enzymes such as amylases and proteases break down large molecules (starch or proteins, respectively) into smaller ones, so they can be absorbed by the intestines. Lipase breaks down fat, cellulase breaks down cellulose (the cell walls of plant fiber).

In 1933, the first enzyme diastase was discovered. Found in the wheat germ, it acts on decomposing the natural starches in the surrounding kernel. By removing both the diastase and the wheat germ, bread had a longer shelf life, however, bread became more difficult to digest. In digestion, enzymes are the active materials within digestive juices that break down the food. Enzymes are keys that unlock nutrients. Enzymes are found in the salivary glands, liver, stomach, pancreas and the wall of the small intestine.

Enzymes are protein molecules that act like spark plugs in the body. Without them we would not survive. For example, ninety-eight enzymes have been found in our arteries. Among these are cytochrome oxidase, peroxidase and catalase, which are components of red and white blood cells. Very high amounts of these enzymes are found in green leafy plants. These enzymes have been shown to destroy toxic substances in the body, therefore, helping protect the body from serious conditions such as cancer.

Enzymes are the biochemical foundation for thousands of digestive and metabolic functions and they are crucial in the healing process. Approximately 5,000 different enzymes have been identified thus far and it is estimated that it more than 100,000 enzymes are required for the body to function properly.

A banana left on the counter for too long becomes over-ripen and turns to mush because of the process of enzymes breaking down and digesting the fruit. In contrast, a bottle of fruit juice can remain fresh for a year because its enzymes have been destroyed by heat in the pasteurization process. Enzymes in living foods are little *digestion machines,* working and assisting to help break down food so that the body may easily assimilate its nutrients. Killing the enzymes for shelf life causes the body to work much harder in digestion and assimilation.

On the other hand, foods such as beef or chicken contain no enzymes to help digestion. The body is forced to produce strong acid secretions to aid digestion along with the help of the pancreas. The pancreas must produce large quantities of proteolytic enzymes which place a heavy burden on it. Eating a high percentage of cooked food on a daily basis causes the pancreas to be chronically over-stimulated, eventually break down. Years and years of such abuse can cause digestive problems such as gastric reflux, gastritis, bloating, gas and constipation.

For optimal health and wellness, all essential nutrients are needed and missing even one can result in seriously breakdown in our health status. When nutrients that are designed to work together have missing members, metabolic processes are disrupted causing cell rebuilding to slow down and aging to speed up. When all nutrients are present, metabolic processes proceed at an ideal rate so that each cell can perform their specific bodily function.

ORGANIC IS THE WAY TO GO

Understanding the magnitude of health hazards makes for an easy decision to purchase organic food over conventionally grown food. More people demand and purchase organic, the more prices will fall and natural or organic will not just be a section in the supermarket.

The methods employed in organic farming differ from conventional farming, in that traditional farmers apply chemical fertilizers to the soil to grow their crops, whereas organic farmers feed and build soil with natural fertilizer. Also, traditional farmers use insecticides to get rid of insects and disease, while organic farmers use natural methods such as insect predators and barriers for this purpose. Conventional farmers control weed growth by applying synthetic herbicides, but organic farmers use crop rotation, tillage, hand weeding, cover crops and mulches to control weeds.

The global sales of organic food are growing in popularity while U.S. organic food sales have increased from $3.5 billion in 1996 to more than $23 billion in 2002.

The result is that conventionally grown food is often tainted with chemical residues, which can be harmful to humans. Any level of chemical contamination should be considered hazardous, especially when the

Environmental Protection Agency (EPA) considers 60 percent of herbicides, 90 percent of fungicides and 30 percent of insecticides to be carcinogenic.

The negative influences of pesticides on health are many, including neurotoxicity, disruption of the endocrine system, carcinogenicity and immune system suppression. Pesticide exposure may also affect male reproductive function and has been linked to miscarriage in women.

Researchers reported that exposure to a mix of two crop-treating chemicals widely used in farming has been linked to Parkinson's disease. The laboratory mice injected with the twin combination of the herbicide Paraquat and the fungicide Maneb showed brain damage identical to humans suffering from Parkinson's. The study found that farmers, rural dwellers and people who drink well water were also more likely to die of Parkinson's disease than people who do not (Agence France Press 04.01.2001, cited from AGNET mail out 04.01.2001).

Another major consideration of conventionally produced foods is the decreased nutrients value compared to organically produced foods. A study published in the Journal of Applied Nutrition 1993; 45:35-39 of organically and conventionally grown apples, potatoes, pears, wheat, and sweet corn analyzed for mineral content yielded the following results. On a per-weight basis, average levels of essential minerals were much higher in the organically grown than in the conventionally grown food. The organically grown food averaged 63% higher in calcium, 78% higher in chromium, 73% higher in iron, 118% higher in magnesium, 178% higher in molybdenum, 91% higher in phosphorus, 125% higher in potassium and 60% higher in zinc. The organically raised food averaged 29% lower in mercury than the conventionally raised food.

On average, conventional produce has only 83 percent of the nutrients of organic produce. Studies have found significantly higher levels of nutrients such as vitamin C, iron, magnesium and phosphorus, and significantly less nitrates (a toxin) in organic crops.

There is no question that organic foods are superior to non-organic produce, however, many people still are not eating any vegetables because they either cannot afford them or they are too difficult to obtain.

Another option is to buy organic produce selectively, as certain foods tend to have higher or lower amounts of pesticides. Try to eat fruits and vegetables with consistently low pesticide loads.

The following foods tend to have the highest levels of pesticides (from Environmental Working Group's Food News):

PESTICIDE LOADS OF FOODS

Most Contaminated	12 Least Contaminated
Apple	Asparagus
Bell Peppers	Avocados
Celery	Bananas
Cherries	Broccoli
Imported Grapes	Cauliflower
Nectarines	Corn(sweet)
Peaches	Kiwi
Pears	Mangos
Potatoes	Onions
Red Raspberries	Papaya
Spinach	Pineapples
Strawberries	Peas (sweet)

What government tests tell us about pesticides in apples, for example, is:

1) Pesticides were found on 91 percent of the apples tested.
2) There were **36 pesticides** <u>found on apples</u>:

> 2 4-d, Acephate, Azinphos methyl, Benomyl, Captan, Carbaryl, Chlorothalonil, Chlorpropham, DDT, Diazinon, Dicloran, Dicofol, Dimethoate, Diphenylamine (DPA), Disulfoton, Endosulfans, Fenbutatin oxide, Fenvalerate, Formetanate hydrochloride, Imazalil, Iprodione, Lindane (BHC gamma), Metalaxyl, Methomyl, Mevinphos Total, Myclobutanil, O-Phenylphenol, Oxamyl, Parathion ethyl, Permethrin Total, Phosalone, Phosmet, Phosphamidon, Propargite, Pyridaben, Thiabendazole

3) The three pesticides found most often on apples were Diphenylamine (DPA), Thiabendazole, and Azinphos methyl.

For more detailed information, visit http://www.foodnews.org/reportcard.php

*** Please understand that it is better to eat non-organic vegetables (locally grown or farmer's markets) than no vegetables at all.

If you must buy conventional produce, there are ways to reduce your pesticide exposure:

✓ Thoroughly washing all fruits and vegetables will help, although all pesticide residues cannot be removed.
✓ You can also remove the outer layer of leaves or peel vegetables if possible.
✓ Another alternative is to grow your own vegetables.

YOUR GUIDE TO EATING

To set the groundwork for a lifestyle of wellness, a criterion for what you choose to eat must be set. ***Eating food cannot be a random act without preparation or forethought.***

GUIDE TO FOOD GROUPS

The most important principles in this series of recommendations are **"Listen to your Body."** If any food or supplement makes you sick in any way, stop it immediately! You have the tools to tell if something is good for your body or not -- please use them!

I. Wellness Plan – The Big Picture

    A. At least one half of your food should be uncooked.

    B. Eat as many fresh vegetables as possible

    C. Eat organically grown food (plant and animal)

    D. Limiting **sugar** is critical to optimal health

    E. Avoid hypoglycemia

    F. Distinguish physical food cravings from emotional food cravings

    G. Drink adequate water daily

II. Food Groups Highlights - Proteins

    A. Proteins are essential for building, maintenance, repair of body tissues

    B. They are major components of our immune system and hormones

    C. Proteins found in all types of food, but not all plants contain complete protein (animal sources do, e.g. meat, eggs, cheese) with the exception of amaranth, buckwheat, hempseed, quinoa, seafood, soybean, spirulina and AFA- a specific type of blue-green algae.

D. Protein intake varies and depends on sex, height, weight and exercise levels

E. Proteins Do's and Don'ts

    1. Check packaged foods for the number of grams of protein per serving

    2. Eggs are an excellent source of protein (Organic eggs).
        a. Don't be afraid of eggs; organic eggs supply a good source of omega-3s and will not increase your bad cholesterol

    3. Restrict your intake of dairy products
        a. If you have allergies, consider avoiding all dairy

    4. Limit or eliminate red meats

    5. Beware of your fish and seafood intake
        a. Mercury and other toxins contamination
        b. The larger the fish, the greater the toxic contamination

    6. Nuts and seeds should be lowered or eliminated, if you have allergies to them
        a. Flaxseeds and walnuts, which can help balance your omega-6 and omega-3
        b. Nut butters with fruit such as apple can be a staple

    7. Watch your bean and legume intake
        a. If you have elevated insulin level.
        b. Symptoms of high insulin levels- Excess weight, Obesity, High cholesterol, High blood pressure

III. Food Groups Highlights - Carbohydrates

Carbohydrates provide fuel for the body in the form of glucose, which is a sugar. There are two types of carbohydrates -- simple and complex. Simple carbohydrates are sugars, such as the ones found in candy, fruits and baked goods. Complex carbohydrates are starches found in beans, nuts, vegetables and whole grains.

Your body prefers the carbohydrates in vegetables rather than grains because it slows the conversion to simple sugars like glucose and decreases your insulin level. On the other hand grain carbohydrates will increase your insulin levels and interfere with your ability to burn fat.

A. Find out your insulin level.
1. Normal fasting blood sugar should be around 87 mg/dL.
2. Fasting blood sugar over 100 suggests insulin resistance
3. Above 100, concerns with respect to future diabetes
4. Diabetes is diagnosed when blood sugar rises above 140 mg/dL.
B. Scale back grains and beans the higher your insulin levels
1. Highly processed food products are not recommended, regardless of insulin level. These include:
    a. Breads, Pasta, Cereal, Bagels, French fries
    b. Chips, Pretzels, Waffles, Pancakes, Baked goods
C. Eat the best vegetables.
1. Red and green leaf lettuce, along with romaine lettuce and spinach, kale, mustard and collard greens, Swiss chards
2. Organic vegetables very important
3. At least 1/2 of your diet should be raw foods, and vegetables
D. Reduce or eliminate your intake of added sweeteners.
1. Avoid sweeteners whenever possible, but the following are acceptable:

a. Agave Nectar, Erythrotol, Stevia, Xylitol

b. Avoid sucrose, high fructose corn syrup(HFCS), Splenda, Nutrasweet, Saccharin

IV. Food Groups Highlights - Fats

Fat is made of fatty acids attached to a substance called glycerol. Fats play an important role in the body; they are essential to build cell membranes, clot blood, absorb vitamins, cushion vital organs and protect us from extreme temperatures.

A. Types of fat

1. **Saturated fats:** found in animal products such as butter, cheese, whole milk, ice cream, cream and fatty meats. Also found in some vegetable oils-namely coconut, palm and palm kernel

2. **Trans-fatty acids:** Fats form when vegetable oil hardens, a process called hydrogenation

a. Can raise LDL (bad cholesterol) levels. They

b. Can also lower HDL (good cholesterol) levels.

3. **Monounsaturated fats:** The best oil is olive oil.

B. Importance of omega-3 and omega-6 fats.

1. Omega-6 fats contribute to insulin and membrane resistance, altering your mood, and impairing learning and cell repair

2. Benefits of omega-3 fats are reduced risk of heart disease, cancer, stroke, Alzheimer's, arthritis and many other degenerative illnesses.

C. Benefits of fish oil found in fish and cod liver oil

1. Helps fight and <u>prevent heart disease, cancer, depression, Alzheimer's, arthritis, diabetes, hyperactivity</u> and <u>many other diseases</u>

2. Increases your energy level and ability to concentrate

3. Provides greater resistance to common illnesses such as flu and cold

D. Omega-3 deficiencies have been tied to the following problems:

1. Mental sharpness on awakening, Depression/well-being

2. Weight gain, Brittle fingernails, Allergies, Arthritis

3. Quality of sleep, Memory problems, Dry hair

4. Dry skin, Concentration, Fatigue

V. Food Groups Highlights - Beverages

Let's start with the most important element of your diet:...**Water!**

Water makes up more than 70 percent of your body's tissues and plays a role in nearly every body function from regulating temperature and cushioning joints to bringing oxygen to the cells and removing waste from the body. Therefore, it's vital to pay attention to what you drink.

A. Drink ½ your weight in ounces of water each day(150 lbs.= 75 ozs)

B. Drink your water at the right pace. (Sip water all day long.)

C. Drink healthy water: spring or purified with 7.2 pH or higher.

1. All municipal water supplies have chlorine and fluorine added.

2. Avoid distilled water- tend to drain your body of minerals.

D. **Avoid all soft drinks!** For every can of soda that a child drinks per day, his or her risk of obesity increases by 60 percent.

PEARL NUMBER FOUR

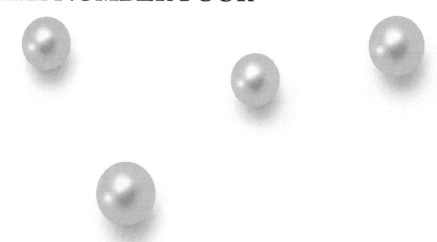

∬ ADDRESS YOUR STRESS ∬

WHAT IS STRESS?

Stress is basically a sudden demand on the body to adapt quickly to a new situation and therefore it depends largely upon perception and sensory input. Stress will thus preoccupy the entire human system whenever it strikes, engaging body, mind and energy in a circle of tension and turmoil if it is not managed well.

Stress that is damaging is created when forces or circumstances outside the body overwhelm the mind, the physiology, and the senses in the body resulting in pathways of negative changes. Studies show a little bit of stress actually can be a good thing. Short-term stress, the type that produces a fight-or-flight response, boosts the immune system, preparing it for possible infection or injury, according to a major review of stress-and-immunity studies in the July 2004 issue of *Psychological Bulletin*, published by the American Psychological Association (APA). But when stress becomes chronic or prolonged, it can wear you down.

149

Unlike the obviously harmful events such as a fresh cut that bleeds, the damaging and even deadly effects of stress can often be a silent killer. There is a direct link between stress and the dysfunction of various parts and systems within the body. Stress reactions alter the digestive system, over-stimulate certain glands while under stimulating others, affect heart function and change breathing. As a result, stress has an actual, measurable negative impact on:

- Blood pressure
- Cholesterol
- Electrolytes
- Brain chemistry
- Blood sugar levels
- Joint function
- Hormonal balance

"In general, we think that anything that lasts longer than a fight or a flight — a few minutes to maybe a few hours — marks the transition from a beneficial to a harmful stress response," said Suzanne C. Segerstrom, an associate professor of psychology at the University of Kentucky in Lexington.

Older people and those who already have compromised immune systems seem to be particularly vulnerable to disease. It does not take years of research and testing to know there is a relationship between stress and disease because of changes in our immune system. It appears to be very apparent in conditions, such as viral cancers and heart disease.

All of the physiological problems associated with stress will speed up the aging process and cause or contribute to literally every type of symptom or disease known to man. Stress even makes you gain weight.

THE PHYSIOLOGY OF STRESS

The human body is equipped to deal with the sort of stress people faced in the pre-industrial world, such as crossing paths with a saber-toothed tiger, tribal warfare, avalanches, floods and other situations that provoke the fight-or-flight response. In such situations, the adrenal glands spurt adrenaline into the bloodstream and switch the nervous system over to the action mode of the sympathetic branch. The body then responds by fighting, running or some other high-energy physical reaction, burning off the simulative hormones and extra glucose pumped into the bloodstream for the purpose, then returning to normal. When such situations occur occasionally and not chronically, they eventually pass and the body naturally recovered its energy and endocrine balance.

Today, the same biochemical responses are triggered, hundreds of times throughout the day and night by frustration in the office, marital strife, repressed rage, bad news on television, exposure to microwaves and abnormal electromagnetic fields, fear alienation, peer pressures and other hazards of modern life. However, instead of making high-energy physical responses, people repress their rage, fear and other negative emotions provoked by stress, thereby failing to utilize the powerful hormones and neurochemicals released into the blood. These potent biochemicals quickly break down into various toxic by-products that poison the system, suppress immunity and impede other vital functions. Under chronic stress, the body never has a chance to excrete these toxins thoroughly and restore proper biochemical balance.

EFFECTS OF CHRONIC STRESS

In recent years, chronic stress has finally become recognized as a major immunosuppressant and a primary cause of dis-ease, especially in the crowded urban centers of industrially developed societies. Stress causes the adrenals to secrete <u>adrenaline</u> and <u>cortisone</u>, the latter being a particularly powerful immunosuppressant, especially in the thymus, lymph nodes and spleen.

Cortisone also impairs production of interferon, one of the body's most potent immunity agents. Diseases associated with high cortisone levels include cancer, hypertension, arthritis, stroke, chronic infections, skin diseases, Parkinson disease and ulcers. The role played by stress in the causation of cancer is so great that it would not be an exaggeration to say that 80% or more cancer cases have their immediate origin in some form of mental pressure or strain.

Grief, distress, fear, worry and anger are emotions which have horrible effects on the body's functions. Researchers have discovered that these emotions cause the release of chemicals from the brain call neuropeptides. These potent compounds have a profound immune-suppressive action.

High levels of anger may help fuel coronary artery disease in many patients under the age of 50, according to researchers. Unresolved emotional and spiritual issues, such as a broken heart, depression, anger or a lack of fulfillment, can physically affect your heart.

According to Dr. Robert O. Young, Director of Research at the pH Miracle Living Center, "anger is energy in motion or E-motion that can require the consumption of a high level of cellular energy and as a result produce a high level of acidic waste that can cause electrical instability in the heart leading to arrhythmia and sudden cardiac arrest."

MORE DATA

Just how stressed-out are we? According to the American Psychological Association's online Help Center:

- Forty-three percent of all adults suffer adverse health effects from stress.
- Seventy-five percent to 90 percent of all physician office visits are for stress-related ailments and complaints.
- Stress is linked to the six leading causes of death — heart disease, cancer, lung ailments, accidents, cirrhosis of the liver, and suicide.

There is plenty of evidence linking stress with premature aging. Researchers at the University of California, San Francisco found that prolonged psychological stress affects molecules that are believed to play a role in cellular aging and, possibly, the onset of disease. In the study, the immune cells of women who care for chronically ill children aged faster than those of women with healthy kids.

STRESS MANAGEMENT

People all face much of the same outside factors that cause stress. Work, relationships, school, personal and family health problems, money issues, and even positive events like weddings and parties can all be stress-producing circumstances. However, none of these things are necessarily bad. Both happy events and tragedies alike cause a stress response in the body. Some stress is unavoidable. The only way to have zero stress is to not get up in the morning!

Stress only becomes <u>negative</u> when your response to it is <u>negative</u>. The condition we call stress is entirely self-induced. It is how each individual responds to stress, and not the stress itself, that causes a negative reaction in the body.

Stress is not a person, a condition or an event. Stress is a reaction to a person, a condition or an event. Just how negative this reaction is will determine the amount of emotional turmoil and damage done to the body. Effectively, any injury induced by stress is a self-inflicted wound.

An example:

Public speaking can cause an amazing amount of negative stress for most people. It scares a lot of people half to death--literally. Then again, public speaking cannot be considered bad stress in and of itself, because while some people are afraid of public speaking and will suffer miserably throughout the entire experience, many others thoroughly enjoy speaking in public and see it as an opportunity to entertain, teach and motivate.

To get to the root of stress you must change the way you look at things. An excellent approach is to make sure to separate anxiety issues from authority issues.

"***Anxiety issues***" are the everyday troubles such as world events, news, professional sports team performance, other people's troubles, and pending personal crisis. Anxiety issues are problems in which you have no direct control over their outcome, yet you nonetheless allow them to create chaos, worry, stress, and a lot of lost time in your own life.

- 40% of our worries will never happen
- 30% of our worries are about the PAST
- 22% of our worries are needless, miscellaneous and petty
- 8% of all our worries are about legitimate concerns

The fact is that worrying is the most useless activity in life. Worrying about the events of the world, other people's lives, or even events in your life does nothing to affect the eventual results. Worrying does nothing but disturb and disrupt what precious few moments we have in this life. Worrying cannot add inch to your life!

Conversely, "**_authority issues_**" are the challenges you can do something about. These are the problems concerning the need for more discipline, more learning, more practicing, better scheduling, improved preparation, etc. There are many instances with people and situations that we have some direct control over. In general, authority issues only concern you, i.e., your actions and reactions are usually the only ones that you can truly totally influence.

If you recognize something as an "authority issue," then you can create a strategy and start actively creating a solution, but if you recognize something as an "anxiety issue," worrying is useless and can create nothing but damaging stress and diminished time.

Live by the scripture Matthew 6:24 which says, *"Therefore do not worry about tomorrow, for tomorrow will worry about itself."*

STRESS SOLUTIONS

Mental factors, such as enthusiasm, are also important in maintaining health. If you are bored or frustrated by your job, hobby, marriage or other activities, your mind lacks enthusiasm for life, which in turn saps the will to live. Simply by changing your habits or creatively solving the problems that frustrate you, you recover enthusiasm, which in turn stimulates vitality and boosts immunity.

Visualization is another effective way to restore immunity and heal the body. Carl and Stephanie Simonton of the Cancer Counseling and Research Center in Dallas, Texas, reported a case of a young boy with cancer to whom they taught a therapeutic method of visualization. Day after day, the boy vividly imagined jet fighters zooming into his body to strafe and bomb his tumors and sure enough, the tumors soon began to shrink and finally disappeared altogether, without chemotherapy, radiation or surgery. Using this technique, the Simontons' have managed to double the survival times of terminal cancer patients under their care.

Meditation is a very effective method for boosting immunity and cultivating the power of positive thinking, visualization and mind over matter. Simply by "sitting still, doing nothing" for a while each day, you give your mind a chance to retire from the stresses of daily life and explore its own innate powers.

Love, although it may sound like a cliché, has great healing powers. The truth is "love heals." Love energizes the entire immune system and specifically stimulates the production of antibodies. Lack of love for oneself and others gives rise to negative thoughts and emotions releases immunosuppressive hormones and neurochemicals into our system.

The Bottom Line: The primary goal is to learn to efficiently manage positive versus negative stress to lessen its effects on our body. First we must change our minds (our thinking). How we view and respond to challenges and circumstances is critical to controlling stress effects on our body.

"Perception is Everything," and our "Response to Perception is Everything Else."

MEASURES TO DE-STRESS

There are a host of measures to de-stress and reduce or even eliminate the damaging effects of stress. Traditional methods include:

1. Relaxation techniques, including meditation, massage and yoga
2. A solid cardiovascular and resistance exercise program will help
3. A good night's sleep — a minimum of seven hours each night
4. Relaxation music tapes with aromatherapy

5. Just walking is very beneficial
6. Don't forget proper nutrition composed of high quality, unprocessed foods.
7. Prayer and spiritual development positively buffers "anxiety issues" and can serve to reduce or even eliminate certain future stresses.

IMPORTANCE OF SLEEP

The human body uses sleep to repair, rebuild and restore itself. In essence, our bodies use the sleeping hours to cleanse and detoxify, and to build strength and immunity. When we eat late at night and go to sleep with a full stomach, the body IS NOT at rest. Even though our mental processes are quiet, our physical body is actually quite busy digesting and processing a large amount of food. This inhibits the vital cleansing, building and restorative processes that normally occur while we sleep. We've all had the experience of going to sleep with a full stomach, and waking the next morning feeling tired, exhausted and disoriented, despite 8 hours of sleep. This is because your body, in actuality, did NOT get 8 hours of sleep... more like 3 hours of sleep, after working hard most of the night to digest and process the big meal you ate before bed. Do not eat late at night! Eat an early dinner, and eat light in the evenings.

SLEEP DO'S AND DON'TS

Here is a list of Do's and Don'ts that can add years to your life and quality to your health. Rome was not built in a day, but the sooner you can adopt all these suggestions, sooner you can experience renewed energy and sense of well-being.

1. **Avoid before-bed snacks, particularly grains and sugars**. This will raise blood sugar and inhibit sleep. Later, when blood sugar drops too low (hypoglycemia), you might wake up and not be able to fall back asleep.

2. **Sleep in complete darkness or as close as possible**. When light hits the eyes, it disrupts the circadian rhythm of the pineal gland and production of melatonin and serotonin. There also should be as little light in the bathroom as possible if you get up in the middle of the night.

3. **No TV right before bed**. Even better, get the TV out of the bedroom or even out of the house, completely. It is too stimulating to the brain and it will take longer to fall asleep. Also disruptive of pineal gland function for the same reason as above.

4. **Read something spiritual or religious**. This will help to relax. Don't read anything stimulating, such as a mystery or suspense novel, as this may have the opposite effect.

5. **Avoid using loud alarm clocks**. It is very stressful on the body to be awoken suddenly. If you are regularly getting enough sleep, they should be unnecessary.

6. **Get to bed as early as possible**. Our systems, particularly the adrenals, do a majority of their recharging or recovering during the hours of 11PM and 1AM. In addition, your gallbladder dumps toxins during this same period. If you are awake, the toxins back up into the liver which then secondarily back up into your entire system and cause further disruption of your health. Prior to the widespread use of electricity, people would go to bed shortly after sundown which nature originally intended for us.

7. **Check your bedroom for electro-magnetic fields (EMFs)**. These can disrupt the pineal gland and the production of melatonin and serotonin, and may have other negative effects as well. Purchase a gauss meter to measure EMFs in your sleep environment. Try the Cutcat at

158

800-497-9516. They have a model for around $40. Dr. Herbert Ross, author of "Sleep Disorders" goes as far as recommending that people pull their circuit breaker before bed to kill all power in their house.

8. **Keep the temperature in the bedroom cooler rather than warmer.** Many people keep their homes and particularly the upstairs bedrooms too hot.

9. **Eat a high-protein snack <u>several hours</u> before bed.** This can provide the L-tryptophan need to produce melatonin and serotonin.

10. **Reduce or avoid as many drugs as possible.** Many medications, both prescription and over-the-counter may have effects on sleep.

11. **Avoid caffeine.** A recent study showed that in some people, caffeine is not metabolized efficiently and therefore they can feel the effects long after consuming it. So an afternoon cup of coffee (or even tea) will keep some people from falling asleep. Also, some medications, particularly diet pills contain caffeine.

12. **Alarm clocks and other electrical devices.** If these devices must be used, keep them as far away from the bed as possible, preferably at least 3 feet.

13. **Avoid alcohol.** Although alcohol will make people drowsy, the effect is short lived and people will often wake up several hours later, unable to fall back asleep. Alcohol will also keep you from falling into the deeper stages of sleep, where the body does most of its healing.

14. **Lose weight.** Being overweight can increase the risk of sleep apnea, which will prevent a restful night's sleep.

15. **Avoid foods that you may be sensitive to.** This is particularly true for dairy and wheat products, as they may have effect on sleep, such as causing apnea, excess congestion, gastrointestinal upset, and gas, among others.

16. **Don't drink any fluids within 2 hours of going to bed.** This will reduce the likelihood of needing to get up and go to the bathroom or at least minimize the frequency.

17. **Take a hot bath, shower or sauna before bed**. When body temperature is raised in the late evening, it will fall at bedtime, facilitating sleep,

18. **Keep Your Bed For Sleeping**. If you are used to watching TV or doing work in bed, you may find it harder to relax and to think of the bed as a place to sleep.

19. **Have your adrenals checked by a good natural medicine clinician**. Scientists have found that Insomnia may be caused by adrenal stress (Journal of Clinical Endocrinology & Metabolism, Aug 2001;86:3787-3794).

BENEFITS OF EXERCISE

How Does Exercise Help?

    Regular exercise lowers blood pressure

    Raises good HDL (good cholesterol)

    Decreases osteoporosis (thinning of the bones)

    Lowers stress/improves depression (releases endorphins)

    Improves circulation

    Helps the pain and stiffness of arthritis

    To fight against aging (losing muscle mass)

Rules for Exercise

    Eat a meal or snack within 1hr prior to exercise

    Do not exercise before bedtime (can lower blood sugar during sleep)

    When possible, check sugar before exercise

    Do not walk up hill/incline, unless Ok'd by your doctor

    Wear comfortable clothes, and proper shoes

Modified Seated Exercise

- o If legs are unstable or you have fallen frequent
- o If it is too painful to stand

PRAYER AND MEDITATION

In 2004, U.S. News & World Report teamed up with BeliefNet, a leading multifaith web site focusing on religion, to collect information about why people pray. Out of 5,600 responses, 1 in 3 said that the most important purpose of prayer was "intimacy with God." Another 28% said the most important purpose of prayer was to "seek God's guidance." While people pray for everything from a cure for cancer to financial issues, most prayers seek to effect super natural changes in circumstances and reflect a desire for a personal relationship with God that is engaging and dynamic.

Prayer is one of the oldest and most effective means of relaxation that humans have. For many, meditation and prayer are quiet inward dialogue that helps them resolve internal conflicts and sort out their troubles. It offers a necessary respite from the world that calms and restores in times of crisis or stress. Whether we sing, write, or speak our prayer, it can be liberating to turn our trust over to God.

Although it is difficult to prove definitively the relationship between prayer and curing disease, many studies have demonstrated the recuperative benefits, both physiological and psychological, of meditation and prayer. It is easy to see how prayer might give us greater optimism, promote faster recovery, allow us to manage stress more effectively, prevent addiction, and assuage feelings of depression and anxiety.

Dr. Dale Matthews, Associate Professor of Medicine at Georgetown University and a practicing physician, has documented the connection between faith and healing. After years of observing and recording the ways his patients benefited from an active spiritual life, Matthews concluded that faith:

- Helps us to stay healthy and avoid life-threatening and disabling diseases such as cancer and heart disease;
- Helps us to recover faster and with fewer complications if they do develop a serious illness;
- Helps us to live longer;
- Helps us to avoid and reduce life-threatening encounters and unanticipated terminal illnesses with greater peacefulness and less pain;
- Helps us to avoid mental illnesses such as depression and anxiety and to cope more effectively with stress;
- Helps us to avoid clear of problems with alcohol, drugs and tobacco;
- Helps us to enjoy a happier marriage and family life;
- Helps us to find a greater sense of meaning and purpose in our lives.

Researchers have found that people who are more involved with religious organizations seem to be able to cope with stress better. According to a joint poll conducted with ABC News and Stanford University, researchers found that prayer worked slightly better than drugs to control pain.

PEARL NUMBER FIVE

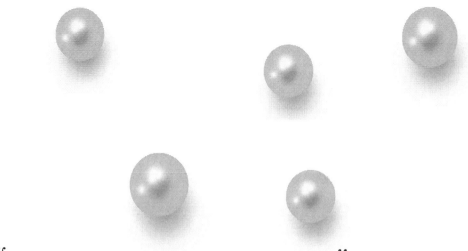

∬ EXTERNAL DETOXIFICATION ∬

WHAT'S ON YOUR BODY?

It is as important to be careful of what we put on our body as what we put in our body. One of the primary sources of toxic chemical exposure is through skin care products and cosmetics. When substance are applied to our skin, up to 40% of them are absorbed directly into the bloodstream. Our skin is not a barrier to most of these chemicals, but actively transports many toxic ingredients directly into our body. The major concern is the accumulative effect of exposing our body to potential and known carcinogens on a daily basis for years. This gradually increasing toxic burden can easy lay the groundwork for disease as well as inhibit the healing processes.

A six-month computer investigation evaluated the safety of over 10,000 personal care product ingredients and included 2,300 people. The investigation revealed the following information on personal care use:

- Each day, **the average adult uses nine personal care products that contain 126 different chemical ingredients**
- Over a quarter of a million women and one out of every 100 men use on the average of 15 products a day

Findings from the Personal Care Safety Assessment

- Only 28 of the 7,500 products in the study were completely tested by the cosmetic industry's self-regulating panel
- An astounding one-third of all the products assessed contained at least one ingredient that fell under the classification of **human carcinogen**
- **71 percent of the hair dye products evaluated had carcinogenic coal tar** as part of their ingredients
- Almost 70 percent of the products reviewed were found to have ingredients that could be tainted with impurities related to cancer and other health complications
- **54 percent of the products violated the safety recommendations** proposed by the self-regulating Cosmetic Ingredient Review Board. Some examples of the unsafe ingredients in these products were discovered in diaper cream, products on the market for damaged skin such as chapped skin and other ingredients found in spray products
- Over the course of keeping watch over the cosmetic industry, the FDA has banned a mere nine personal care products

Based on these findings, researchers agreed that the lack of monitoring by the FDA has led to a huge leniency toward the testing of cosmetic ingredients and has resulted in a large portion of products available on the market that pose health risks to the consumers.

The most common reactions to the chemicals are eczema, psoriasis and dermatitis. However, there is evidence that people who work with these chemicals (such as hairdressers and beauticians) suffer from the cumulative effects of the chemical. The studies concluded that:

- There is an increased risk of lung, uterine, ovarian, breast, digestive and respiratory cancer.

- Of the 169 permanent hair dyes, 150 are mutagenic (cause changes to our cells genes).

- The use of permanent and semi-permanent hair dyes is associated with increased risk of non-Hodgkin's lymphoma, multiple myeloma, leukemia and Hodgkin's disease.

The ingredients that you need to avoid include:

- **Foaming agents** including sodium laureth sulphate (SLS), ammonium lauryl sulphate and 1, 4-dioxane.

- **Artificial fragrances** - many chemicals are able to gain access to our body via our olfactory system or sublingually (under the tongue). In the case of toothpaste a single fragrance can be made up of 200 chemicals which don't have to be labeled. Many fragrances are based on petroleum products and some reactions to these include dizziness, skin irritation and brown tinges to the skin. Products that are fragranced with essential oils are your safest choices.

- **Artificial colors** - things have improved since Queen Elizabeth 1 died from lead poisoning caused by her trademark white make up. However, there are still many questionable colorants. Synthetic colors are made up from coal tar containing heavy metal salts that deposit toxins into our systems.

- **Emulsifiers** - these are used in just about all personal grooming products. They keep the texture uniform and stop the ingredients from separating. Eggs can be used for this but skin care companies prefer a more synthetic version. Glyceryl monostearate and stearic acid are two commonly used emulsifiers and oral care products that are known to cause side effects - in particular skin irritations. Another commonly used emulsifier is triethanolamine, a substance that is converted in living tissue into nitrosamines - some of the strongest carcinogens known. Triethanolamine causes skin irritation problems. Ethoxylates is another commonly used emulsifier which is a strongly mutagenic. It damages the DNA which increases skin aging and the risk of developing skin cancers.

- **Preservatives** - These are used to slow the rate at which the products decay and therefore increase the products shelf life. Some of these that need to be avoided are:

- **Imidazolidinyl urea** - formaldehyde. This is known to cause dermatitis, skin irritation, nerve damage and cancers.

- **Parabens** - over 90% of cosmetics contain a preservative from the parabens family. Some of the latest research suggests that these may work as endocrine disruptors. These chemical play a role in increasing the rate of breast cancer and decreasing rates of male fertility.

- **Carrying agents** - this is the ingredient that provides all the other ingredients a means to be suspended. Water is the most common carrying agent and some are derived from vegetable glycerine or seaweed. However, it is usually a petroleum derivative.

- **Propylene glycol** is commonly used and there are general warnings about it when it is in contact with the skin. It can cause brain, liver and kidney problems. Yet this is the agent that is commonly used in stick deodorants, toothpaste and most other personal care items!

- Other ingredients to watch out for are PVP/VA copolymer, stearalkonium chloride, petrolatum and paraffin.

Skin and hair care products are used in an attempt to enhance our appearance or preserve our skin - however this is not what many of the products that are commercially available actually do. Many are far from safe and add to the toxic burden of the body.

PERSONAL CARE SOLUTIONS

The primary rule of thumb is **"DO NOT PUT ANYTHNG ON YOUR SKIN THAT YOU CANNOT EAT."** Any personal care items that are designed to moisturize, lubricate, cleanse or condition should be from nontoxic, edible sources, and not from unknown chemical or toxic sources. Forty percent of whatever substance that is put on our skin is absorbed into our bloodstream. The concern is with the accumulative effect of daily applications of toxic ingredients to our body and thereby entering our internal environment. We know transdermal and sublingual absorption are effective means to get medications into our bodies so we must seriously guard against physical pollution. If you cannot eat it, do not put it on your body. Here are some very practical solutions:

A. **For skin and hair care –**
  a. For bathing, use chemical-free, fragrance-free, natural bar or liquid soaps made with organic oils and essential oils such as Dr. Bronner's bar and castile soap products.
  b. There is only one true "moisturizer" on the earth which is water. Since our body is 65-70% water, it is the one basic ingredient for

167

soft, supple skin as well as a healthy body. After a bath or shower, apply Shea butter, olive oil or coconut oil to hold moisture in our skin.

c. Do not use petroleum jelly products for feet, knees, elbows, lips or hair. Using natural butters (shea or coco), jojoba oil, grapeseed oil, eucalyptus oil, etc. is the simplest and safest way to maintain healthy skin. It is also extremely economically compared to purchasing expensive, toxic chemicals diluted in water.

d. Use 100% organic soaps such as Dr. Bronner bar and castile soaps free of artificial colors and fragrances. African Black soap and MSM soap are excellent for addressing acne and oily or sensitive skin.

e. In place of synthetic chemical "fragrances," use natural or organic essential oils. Many perfumes and colognes have powerful odors that tend to irritate the nose and eyes and provoke sneezing or coughing. Essential oils tend not to have an overbearing odor but are pleasant and have soothing, relaxing or stimulating qualities. Again, it's all about safety and prevention of potential health challenges. (See Fragrance Analysis in Appendix III).

f. In place of antiperspirants, simply use baking soda lightly applied to underarms or mineral salts rocks. These options eliminate offensive odors, but do not inhibit perspiration. Perspiring is the healthiest and most natural form of body detoxification. When it is prevented, we only increase our toxic burden and risk for chronic illness.

g. Please use natural insect repellant with citronella or other herbal oil bases as opposed to products with DEET (N, N-Diethyl-m-toluamide). DEET can be very harmful to adults and children, is a known eye irritant and may cause rashes, soreness or blistering when applied to the skin. DEET has been linked to neurological problems in adults and children over the decades.

B. For oral hygiene –

a. Toothpaste should be from all natural ingredients and not latent with chemical cleansers and whiteners. Do not put any products in your mouth that has a hazardous warning label on the packaging.

b. Use oil of peppermint for breath freshening, not mint candies full of sugars or artificial sweeteners. If your mouthwash has a "poisoning warning" on the package, do not use it.

c. Poor dental hygiene is directly related to increased risk for cardiovascular disease. Flossing daily to remove plaque is one of the most important prevention activities one can do to maintain optimal health. Even more effect, is the use of a Waterpik to remove plaque along with regular brushing to clean teeth and gums.

DETOXIFYING YOUR HOME ENVIRONMENT

Use Natural Alternatives or Purchase Non-Toxic, Eco-Friendly Household Products

Many conventional cleaning products are petroleum-based and chemically-laden with known carcinogens. Not only are these products a hazard when they come in contact with your skin, but the "off-gassing" of fumes from these chemical compounds pose it own serious challenge to your health (See product chart).

COMMON HOUSEHOLD CLEANING PRODUCTS

Product	Chemical	Reaction
Toilet Bowl Cleaner	Chlorinated Phenol	Toxic to Respiratory & Cardiovascular Systems
Window Cleaners	Diethylene Glycol	Depresses Nervous System
Disinfectants	Phenols	Toxic to Respiratory & Cardiovascular Systems
Laundry Detergents	Nonyl Phenol Ethoxylate	Biodegrades slowly to a toxin
Spray Deodorizers	Formaldehyde	Respiratory Irritant / Carcinogen
Floor Cleaners	Petroleum	Damages Mucous Membranes
Stain Remover	Perchloroethylene	Liver & Kidney Damage
All Purpose Cleaners	Butyl Cellosolve	Damages Bone Marrow, Nervous System, Kidneys, & Liver

Begin by reducing or eliminating these items from underneath your cabinets and in your pantry. Here are a few natural and economical substitutes:

- *Replace traditional glass cleaners with white vinegar.* It works just as well, and leaves behind a fresh (not vinegary) smell. It's also a natural deterrent to fungi and bacteria.

- *Replace conventional abrasive cleaners with baking soda and lemon juice.* And instead of drinking that acidic cola soft drink, let it go flat and pour it into the toilet as a great bowl cleanser.

- *Create your own insect repellent that doesn't contain harmful insecticides.* Spraying your lawn with chemical pesticides exposes your children and your pets to high levels of toxins - because they are smaller, they have less of a defense against them. There are better ways to eliminate household pests. For ants and cockroaches, try a potent blend of crushed garlic, onion, red pepper, soap, and hot water. Let the mixture sit for a couple of days, then strain before using. Many other insects, such as spiders and beetles, are completely harmless. Instead of killing them, gently move them outside.

- *Replace furniture and shoe polishes with olive oil or a blend of almond and baby oil.* It smells great and brings out a brilliant shine in both leather and natural wood.

- *Disinfect multiple surfaces with a blend of citricidal or tea tree oil and water.* Add 20 drops of citricidal or up to 50 drops of tea tree oil (found at most health food stores) to a bucket of water. Stir well. Use this for wiping floors, counters, sinks, bathroom tiles, shower stalls, and toilet seats. A few drops of citricidal mixed with water will also discourage mold growth in shower stalls. Spray directly on tile.

These are just a few of the alternatives you can try. As you may have noticed, many of these are inexpensive items most people keep in their homes. You'll save money and improve your health at the same time. For bio-friendly household products, see www.healthyhome.com or similar websites.

THE AIR YOU BREATHE

A recent EPA study indicated that the air in homes has chemical contamination levels 70 times greater than outdoor air. This is because houses retain contaminants longer than outside air. So open your windows and doors as often as weather permits, and keep a regular flow of air circulating with ceiling and exhaust fans. Remember--a lot of clutter in your house will inhibit the flow of air and make it more difficult to clean the house thoroughly. The more accumulated junk you have, the more toxic your home, as these items often collect dust, mold, and bacteria.

Other air purification tips:

- Remove wall-to-wall carpeting (few things are more toxic than carpets, as they collect dust, lint, mold, and outdoor toxins and bacteria brought in by shoes). Hardwood floors with a non-toxic varnish are very attractive and a lot healthier. To reduce noise, use organic hemp or cotton area rugs that can be frequently laundered.

- Dehumidify the basement.
- Repair roof and foundation cracks that cause moisture build-up in the home.
- Purchase a high-quality air filter (see www.allerair.com or www.iqair.com)
- Perform regular maintenance checks on your furnace and fireplaces.
- Buy house plants that remove chemicals from the air naturally, such as English Ivy, Peace Lily, or Spider plants.

CLOSING THOUGHTS

> *Dear friend, I pray that you may enjoy good health and that all may go well with you, even as your soul is getting along well.* - *3 John 2*

∬ YOUR BEGINNING ∬

The information shared with you in this book only answers the question, "Where do I start to change my lifestyle"? Wellness is a journey and not a destination. In other words, each day is another opportunity to institute changes to enhance our well-being. It is analogous to us working everyday in our professions to improve our station in life, only this focus is on spiritual and physical body.

We must always keep in mind the big picture, that is, to "prevent or defeat" chronic illness and disease. Our world in 2010 suggests that it is not a question of "if" we confront a serious health challenge, but "when" we will face a challenge. This prospective dictates that it is imperative to be proactive about our health status rather than waiting for the shoe to drop. We are up against a healthcare system that has evolved into a machine whose major concern is managing disease, rather than eliminating it. Medicine today is mainly about treating symptoms or just putting band-aids on problems and never addressing the root cause of an imbalance.

The bottom line is to realize and act on the fact that we hold the primary responsibility for our health, not the doctor, our healthcare system, our insurer or the pharmaceutical company. We cannot remain uninformed about the causes or preventive measures to avoid disease. Re-educating ourselves is an ongoing process and you cannot rely on what was fact even five years ago.

The paradigm shift in health care is more than just trying to eat better and have a healthier lifestyle, but living a life based on prevention rather than treatment. The foundation of our entire healthcare system is currently based around the "emergency room" because treatment and disease management is what pays. This approach lulls us into a mindset whereas we do not address health issues or even realize we have a problem until we end up in the emergency room.   We must design a life plan that establishes, "a case for prevention" first, then "in case of emergency." Again, prevention is the key to eliminating 85% of all sickness and disease.

The foundation of optimal health is to follow these "Five Pearls of Prevention":

1) Internal Detoxification
2) Build Immunity
3) Correct Nutrition Choices
4) Manage Stress
5) External Detoxification

My hope and prayer is that this book will be a benefit and a blessing to you, the reader and everyone you touch.

PREVENTION IS THE KEY!

APPENDICES

APPENDIX I

FOOD COLOR ADDITIVES

Number	Name	Comments
E102	Tartrazine	FD&C Yellow No.5; known to provoke asthma attacks (though the US FDA** do not recognize this) and urticaria (nettle rash) in children (the US FDA** estimates 1:10 000); also linked to thyroid tumours, chromosomal damage, urticaria (hives) and hyperactivity; tartrazine sensitivity is also linked to aspirin sensitivity; used to colour drinks, sweets, jams, cereals, snack foods, canned fish, packaged soups; banned in Norway and Austria
E104	Quinoline Yellow	FD&C Yellow No.10; used in lipsticks hair products, colognes; also in a wide range of medications; cause dermatitis; banned in USA and Norway
E110#	Sunset Yellow FCF, Orange Yellow S	FD&C Yellow No.6; used in cereals, bakery, sweets, snack foods, ice cream, drinks and canned fish; synthetic; also in many medications including Polaramine, Ventolin syrup; side effects are urticaria (hives), rhinitis (runny nose), nasal congestion, allergies, hyperactivity, kidney tumours, chromosomal damage, abdominal pain, nausea and vomiting, indigestion, distaste for food; seen increased incidence of tumours in animals; banned in Norway
E122	Azorubine, Carmoisine	red colour; coal tar derivative; can produce bad reactions in asthmatics and people allergic to aspirin; typical products are confectionary, marzipan, jelly crystals; banned in Sweden, USA, Austria and Norway
E123	Amaranth	FD&C Red No.2; derived from the small herbaceous plant of the same name; used in cake mixes, fruit-flavoured fillings, jelly crystals; can provoke asthma, eczema and hyperactivity; it caused birth defects and fetal deaths in some animal tests, possibly also cancer; banned in the USA, Russia, Austria and Norway and other countries
E124	Ponceau 4R,	FD&C Red No.4; synthetic coal tar and azo dye, carcinogen in

	Cochineal Red A	animals, can produce bad reactions in asthmatics and people allergic to aspirin; banned in USA & Norway
E127	Erythrosine	FD&C Red No.3; red colour used in cherries, canned fruit, custard mix, sweets, bakery, snack foods; can cause sensitivity to light; can increase thyroid hormone levels and lead to hyperthyroidism, was shown to cause thyroid cancer in rats in a study in 1990; banned in January 1990, but not recalled by the US FDA**; banned in Norway
E128	Red 2G	Banned in Australia and many other places except UK
E129	Allura red AC	FD&C Red No.40; Orange-red colour used in sweets, drinks and condiments, medications and cosmetics, synthetic; introduced in the early eighties to replace amaranth which was considered not safe due to conflicting test results; allura red has also been connected with cancer in mice; banned in Denmark, Belgium, France, Germany, Switzerland, Sweden, Austria and Norway
E132#	Indigotine, Indigo carmine	FD&C Blue No.2, commonly added to tablets and capsules; also used in ice cream, sweets, baked goods, confectionary, biscuits, synthetic coal tar derivative; may cause nausea, vomiting, high blood pressure, skin rashes, breathing problems and other allergic reactions. Banned in Norway
E133	Brilliant blue FCF	FD&C Blue Dye No.1; used in dairy products, sweets and drinks, synthetic usually occurring as aluminum lake (solution) or ammonium salt; banned in Belgium, France, Germany, Switzerland, Sweden, Austria, Norway
E140	Chlorophylis, Chlorophyllins	green colour occurs naturally in all plants; used for dyeing waxes and oils, used in medicines and cosmetics
E142	Green S	green colour; synthetic coal tar derivative; used in canned peas, mint jelly and sauce, packet bread crumbs and cake mixes; banned in Sweden, USA and Norway
E150(a)	Plain caramel	dark brown colour made from sucrose; the HACSG* recommends to avoid it. used in oyster, soy, fruit and canned sauces, beer, whiskey, biscuits, pickles
E151	Brilliant Black	color; coal tar derivative; used in brown sauces, black currant

179

	BN, Black PN	cake mixes; banned in Denmark, Belgium, France, Germany, Switzerland, Sweden, Austria, USA, Norway
E153#	Vegetable carbon	black colour, charcoal pigment; used in jams, jelly crystals, liquorice; only the vegetable derived variety permitted in Australia, banned in the United States
E155	Brown HT (Chocolate)	brown colour, coal tar and azo dye; used in chocolate cake mixes; can produce bad reactions in asthmatics and people allergic to aspirin; also known to induce skin sensitivity; banned in Denmark, Belgium, France, Germany, Switzerland, Sweden, Austria, USA, Norway
E160(a)#	Carotene, alpha-, beta-, gamma-	orange-yellow colour; human body converts it to 'Vitamin A' in the liver, found in carrots and other yellow or orange fruits and vegetables
E160(b)#	Annatto (Arnatto, Annato), bixin, norbixin	red colour; derived from a tree (Bixa orellana); used as a body paint, fabric dye, digestive aid and expectorant; used to dye cheese, butter, margarine, cereals, snack foods, soaps, textiles and varnishes; known to cause urticaria (nettle rash), the HACSG* recommends to avoid it
E160(c)#	Paprika extract, capsanthin, capsorubin	avoid it, banned in some countries
E160(d)#	Lycopene	red coloured carotenoid found in tomatoes and pink grapefruit, can cause decreasing risk of cancer

* Hyperactive Children Support Group (HACSG)

** Food and Drug Administration

Additives which are probably or definitely animal (mostly pig) derivation.

. This list is adapted from http://www.additives.8m.com/english.htm

APPENDIX II

Safe Harbor - Find safe alternatives at any of the following stores.

The Container Store   www.containerstore.com   888.266.8246
Offers a broad selection, including Stackable Square Glass Canisters

Crate and Barrel   www.crateandbarrel.com   800.967.6696
Look for the Storage Bowl set or the Refrigerator Dishes ($5.95-$7.95/each).

Ball Mason Jars   www.ballmasonjars.biz   877.880.8877
Inexpensive and sturdy, the half-pint jars are ideal for packing kids' school-lunch snacks (about $8-$12 for 12).

Stainless Steel Thermos www.thermos.com   800.243.0745
A range of stainless-steel containers for beverages and edibles.

Classic Glass Nurser Bottles www.lansinoh.com   800.292.4794
Lansinoh Breastmilk Storage Bottles - fits on breast pump.

APPENDIX III

- Analysis Summary -
Calvin Klein's *Eternity eau de parfum*

Calvin Klein's *Eternity eau de parfum*

What you think you are buying:

> "A romantic floral fragrance. Freesia, mandarin and sage accent the top note which combines with muguet, white lily, marigold and narcissus from the white floral bouquet that is the middle note. Patchouli with exotic notes of sandalwood and amber complete the background." ***The Fragrance Foundation 2002 Reference Guide,*** page 185. *Eternity* was created by the Calvin Klein Cosmetics Company in 1988. UNILEVER COSMETICS INTERNATIONAL

What you are buying:
See Analysis Summary Below:

Chemical information acquired via MSDS:
    Aldrich (http://www.sigmaaldrich.com)

    Fisher Chemical MSDS at (https://www2.fishersci.com/chemical/info/msdsinfo.jsp)

    EPA's Toxic Substances Control Act (TSCA) Inventory
(http://msds.pdc.cornell.edu/tscasrch.asp). Also, see below.

    Registry of Toxic Effects of Chemical Substances. (RTECS)
(http://www.cdc.gov/niosh/rtecs.html). Also, see below.

    Search RTECS Database: (http://ccinfoweb.ccohs.ca/rtecs/search.html)

Chemical	CAS# Chemical Abstracts Service A unique number assigned to every individually identifiable substance.	**Reference Material** Searches conducted by CAS number. You must register to access MSDS information, then click on MSDS and do a search for the chemical. Visit: **Aldrich** and **Fisher** are linked to those sites. To see listed on *Registry of Toxic Effects of Chemical Substances*, visit **Search RTECS Database** To query the *Toxic Substances Control Act (TSCA) Chemical Substances Inventory,* visit **Cornell**

Hydrocinnamaldehyde, p-tert-butyl-.alpha.-methyl- **(Lilial)**	80-54-6	Irritant. The chemical, physical, and toxicological properties have not been thoroughly investigated. Label Precautions: **TARGET ORGAN DATA: BEHAVIORAL (SOMNOLENCE) [drowsiness]; LUNGS, THORAX OR RESPIRATION (DYSPNAE) [difficulty breathing]; PATERNAL EFFECTS (TESTES, EPIDIDYMIS, SPERM DUCT)** (<u>Aldrich</u>) Listed: **Registry of Toxic Effects of Chemical Substances.**
Benzoic acid, 2-hydroxy-, phenylmethyl ester **(Benzyl Salicylate)**	118-58-1	Irritant. The chemical, physical, and toxicological properties have not been thoroughly investigated. (<u>Aldrich</u>) (<u>Fisher</u>) Listed: **Registry of Toxic Effects of Chemical Substances.**
Phthalic acid, diethyl ester **(Diethyl Phthalate)**	84-66-2	Irritant, CNS effects, may cause fetal effects. (<u>Aldrich</u>) (<u>Fisher</u>) Listed: **Registry of Toxic Effects of Chemical Substances.** **#TI1050000.** http://www.cdc.gov/niosh/rtecs/ti100590.html
3-Cyclohexene-1-methanol, alph.,.alpha.,4-trimethyl-	98-55-5	Irritant. The chemical, physical, and toxicological properties have not been thoroughly investigated. (<u>Aldrich</u>) (<u>Fisher</u>) Listed: **Registry of Toxic Effects of Chemical Substances.**
1,3-Benzodioxole- 5-carboxaldehyde	120-57-0	Irritant, CNS effects The chemical, physical, and toxicological properties have not been thoroughly investigated. (<u>Aldrich</u>) (<u>Fisher</u>)
Cyclopenta(g) -2-benzopyran, 1,3,4,6,7,8-hexadro- 4,6,6,7,8-hexamethyl- (GALAXOLIDE 50) -- a	1222-05-5	"Irritant ... TOXICOLOGICAL INFORMATION: Acute effects: To the best of our knowledge, the chemical, physical, and toxicological properties have not been thoroughly investigated.

183

synthetic musk compound, "fluidized with diethyl phthalate" (IFF)		Causes skin irritation. May be harmful if absorbed through the skin. May cause eye irritation. May be harmful if inhaled. Material may be irritating to mucous membranes and upper respiratory tract. May be harmful if swallowed. <u>Hazardous ingredients: Contains diethyl phthalate,</u> chemical abstracts registry number 84-66-2. (**Aldrich**)
Benzoic acid, 2-hydroxy-, (3Z)-3-hexenyl ester	65405-77-8	Irritant. The chemical, physical, and toxicological properties have not been thoroughly investigated. [May be harmful by inhalation, ingestion, skin absorption. Vapor or mist is irritating to the eyes, mucous membranes and upper respiratory tract. causes skin irritation. (**Aldrich**)
1,6-Nonadien-3-ol, 3,7-dimethyl-	10339-55-6	AKA Ethyl Linalool; info not available through Aldrich. From Givaudan: Ethyl Linalool has a lavender, bergamot, coriander character and is more floral, sweeter and less agrestic than Linalool. As with Linalool, it is used in a wide variety of notes for floral bouquets. Tenacity on blotter: 12 hours. http://ingredients.givaudan.com/appl/ fib/ing.nsf/0c7c7a0c6b30d410c1256913002ed09f/ 3f47c12fb093ea4bc1256a380030922e?OpenDocument
6-Octen-1-ol, 3,7-dimethyl-	106-22-9	Severe Irritant. The chemical, physical, and toxicological properties have not been thoroughly investigated. (**Aldrich**) (**Fisher**).
3-Buten-2-one, 4-(2,6,6-trimethyl-2-cyclohexen-1-yl)-	127-41-3	Irritant, skin & respiratory sensitizer. The chemical, physical, and toxicological properties have not been thoroughly investigated. (**Aldrich**)
Acetic acid, phenylmethyl ester	140-11-4	Toxic. May cause CNS effects, irritant, may cause cancer based upon animal studies. The chemical, physical, and toxicological properties have not been thoroughly investigated. (**Aldrich**) (**Fisher**)

Octanol, -hydroxy-3,7-dimethyl-	107-75-5	Irritant. The chemical, physical, and toxicological properties have not been thoroughly investigated. (**Aldrich**) (**Fisher**)
Benzene ethanol	60-12-8	Toxic, harmful by all routes, readily absorbed via skin, CNS effects. (**Aldrich**) Listed: **Registry of Toxic Effects of Chemical Substances.** as "Phenethyl alcohol." .
Phenol, 2-methoxy-4-(1-propenyl)-	97-54-1	Irritant. The chemical, physical, and toxicological properties have not been thoroughly investigated. (**Aldrich**)
2-Propen-1-ol, 3-phenyl-	104-54-1	Irritant. The chemical, physical, and toxicological properties have not been thoroughly investigated. (**Aldrich**) (**Fisher**) Listed: **Registry of Toxic Effects of Chemical Substances.** as "Cinnamyl alcohol."
7-Octen-4-one, 2,6-dimethyl-	1879-00-1	No records found as of 11/03/02.
Phenol, 2,6-bis(1,1-dimethylethyl)-4-methyl-	128-37-0	Irritant, cancer suspect agent, may cause reproductive/fetal effects The chemical, physical, and toxicological properties have not been thoroughly investigated. (**Aldrich**) (**Fisher**)
Benzene methanol	100-51-6	Irritant, skin sensitizer, CNS effect, harmful by all routes of exposure. (**Aldrich**) (**Fisher**) Listed: **Registry of Toxic Effects of Chemical Substances.** as "Benzyl alcohol."
Benzoic acid, 2-hydroxy-, ethyl ester	118-61-6	Irritant. The chemical, physical, and toxicological properties have not been thoroughly investigated. (**Aldrich**) (**Fisher**)

Updated 11/03/02 with links to TSCA and RTECS

Background: TSCA -- Toxic Substance Control Act, as amended
By *ChemAlliance.org*"

... A major objective of TSCA is to characterize and evaluate the risks posed by a chemical to humans and the environment before the chemical is introduced into commerce. TSCA accomplishes this through the requirement that manufacturers perform various kinds of health and environmental testing, use quality control in their production processes, and notify EPA of information they gain on possible adverse health effects from use of their products. Under TSCA, "manufacturing" is defined to include "importing", and thus all requirements applicable to manufacturers apply to importers as well.

"EPA has authority to ban the manufacture or distribution in commerce, limit the use, require labeling, or place other restrictions on chemicals that pose unreasonable risks. Among the chemicals EPA regulates under TSCA are asbestos, chlorofluorocarbons (CFCs), and polychlorinated biphenyls (PCBs). ..."

http://www.chemalliance.org/Handbook/background/back-tsca.asp

Registry of Toxic Effects of Chemical Substances (RTECSÆ)
By *Thomson Dialog*"

The Registry of Toxic Effects of Chemical Substances (RTECSÆ) is a comprehensive database of basic toxicity information for over 100,000 chemical substances including: prescription and non-prescription drugs, food additives, pesticides, fungicides, herbicides, solvents, diluents, chemical wastes, reaction products of chemical waste, and substances used in both industrial and household situations. Reports of the toxic effects of each compound are cited. In addition to toxic effects and general toxicology reviews, data on skin and/or eye irritation, mutation, reproductive consequences and tumorigenicity are provided. Federal standards and regulations, NIOSH recommended exposure limits and information on the activities of the EPA, NIOSH, NTP, and OSHA regarding the substance are also included. The toxic effects are linked to literature citations from both published and unpublished governmental reports, and published articles from the scientific literature. The database corresponds to the print version of the Registry of Toxic Effects of Chemical Substances, formerly known as the Toxic Substances List started in 1971, and is prepared by the National Institute for Occupational Safety and Health (NIOSH).

"Toxicity information appearing in RTECS is derived form reports of acute, chronic, lethal and non-lethal effects of chemical substances. The reviewed information from the scientific literature and published governmental reports plus unpublished test data from the EPA TSCA test submissions database (TSCATS) are included in the file.

"http://library.dialog.com/bluesheets/html/bl0336.html

BIBLIOGRAPHY

BIBLIOGRAPHY

American Cancer Society (December 2007). "Report sees 7.6 million global 2007 cancer deaths". Reuters. http://www.reuters.com/article/healthNews/idUSN1633064920071217. Retrieved on 2008-08-07.

Food, Nutrition, Physical Activity, and the Prevention of Cancer: a Global Perspective. World Cancer Research Fund (2007). ISBN 978-0-9722522-2-5. *Full text*

Le Marchand L, Hankin JH, Bach F, et al. An ecological study of diet and lung cancer in the South Pacific. Int J Cancer 1995 Sep 27; 3(1):18-23.

Merlo LM, Pepper JW, Reid BJ, Maley CC (December 2006). "Cancer as an evolutionary and ecological process". *Nat. Rev. Cancer* **6** (12): 924–35. doi:10.1038/nrc2013. PMID 17109012.

Parkin D, Bray F, Ferlay J, Pisani P (2005). "Global cancer statistics, 2002". *CA Cancer J Clin* **55** (2): 74–108. doi:10.3322/canjclin.55.2.74. PMID 15761078. http://caonline.amcancersoc.org/cgi/content/full/55/2/74.

Robert A. Weinberg (September 1996) (PDF). *How Cancer Arises; An explosion of research is uncovering the long-hidden molecular underpinnings of cancer—and suggesting new therapies.* pp. 62–70. http://www.bme.utexas.edu/research/orly/teaching/BME303/Weinberg.pdf. "Introductory explanation of cancer biology in layman's language".

WHO (February 2006). "Cancer". World Health Organization. http://www.who.int/mediacentre/factsheets/fs297/en/. Retrieved on 2007-06-25.

Wu HT, Lin SH, Chen YH. Inhibition of cell proliferation and in vitro markers of angiogenesis by indole-3-carbinol, a major indole metabolite present in cruciferous vegetables. J Agric Food Chem 2005:53(13):5164-5169.

Xiao D, Srivastava SK, Lew KL, et al. Allyl isothiocyanate a constituent of cruciferous vegetables inhibits proliferation of human prostate cancer cells by causing G2/M arrest and inducing apoptosis. Carcinogenesis 2003;24(5):891-897.

FOOD and NUTRITION

Anon. Vitamin D supplement in early childhood and risk for Type I (insulin-dependent) diabetes mellitus. The EURODIAB Substudy 2 Study Group. Diabetologia. 1999 Jan;42(1):51-4.

Cannell JJ, Vieth R, Umhau J,C et al. Epidemic influenza and vitamin D. Epidemiol Infect. 2006 Dec;134(6):1129-40.

Cantorna MT, Mahon BD. D-hormone and the immune system. J Rheumatol Suppl. 2005 Sep;76:11-20.

Jeannine Delwiche (2004). "The impact of perceptual interactions on perceived flavor". *Food Quality and Preference* **15**: 137–146.

Jeffrey M. Smith (2007). "Seeds of Deception: Exposing Industry and Government Lies About the Safety of the Genetically Engineered Foods You're Eating".

Kiefer D. Unraveling a centuries-old mystery. Why is flu risk so much higher in the winter? Life Extension. February, 2007:228.

Mattes JA, Gittelman R (1981). "Effects of artificial food colorings in children with hyperactive symptoms. A critical review & results of a controlled study". *Arch Gen Psychiatry* **38** (6):714–718.

Pozzilli P, Manfrini S, Crino A, et al. Low levels of 25-hydroxyvitamin D3 and 1,25-dihydroxyvitamin D3 in patients with newly diagnosed type 1 diabetes. Horm Metab Res. 2005 Nov;37(11):680-3.

TJ David (1987). "Reactions to dietary tartrazine". *Archives of Disease in Childhood* **62**: 119–122.

"Vegetarian Diets". United States Department of Agriculture.

ELETROMAGNETIC FREQUENCY

ELF: Extremely Low Frequency, usually the electrical power frequencies of either 60Hz or 50Hz. Assessment of Health Effects from Exposure to Power-Line Frequency Electric and Magnetic Fields, Section 5.1, page 411, NIEHS Working Group Report, National Institute of Environmental Health Sciences of the National Institutes of Health, August 1998.

Kheifets, et al.; Occupational Electric and Magnetic Field Exposure and Brain Cancer: A MetaAnalysis; Journal of Occupational and Environmental Medicine, Vol. 37, No. 12, December 1995, 13271340.

Microwave News, July/August 2001, Page 1.

Paul Brodeur; Currents of Death; Power Lines, Computer Terminals and the Attempt to Cover Up Their Threat to Your Health; Simon and Schuster, 1989.

Sadlonova J, et al.; The effect of the pulsatile electromagnetic field in children suffering from bronchial asthma. Acta Physiol Hung. 2003;90(4):327-34 [Slovakia]

Speers, et al.; Occupational exposures and brain cancer mortality: a preliminary study of East Texas residents. Am J Ind Med. 1988; 13: 629-638.

ONLINE ARTICLES

1. <u>Agriculture and Food—Agricultural Production Indices: Food production per capita index</u>, World Resources Institute

2. <u>2008: The year of global food crisis</u>

3. <u>Food crisis will take hold before climate change, warns chief scientist</u>

4. <u>Global food crisis looms as climate change and fuel shortages bite</u>

5. <u>Experts: Global Food Shortages Could 'Continue for Decades'</u>

6. <u>Has Urbanization Caused a Loss to Agricultural Land?</u>

7. <u>The World's Growing Food-Price Crisis</u>

8. <u>The cost of food: Facts and figures</u>

9. <u>Feed the world? We are fighting a losing battle, UN admits</u>

10. <u>New ISPP Journal.</u> *Food Security: The Science, Sociology and Economics of Food Production and Access to Food*

11. "<u>Food Security in the United States: Measuring Household Food Security</u>" (HTML). USDA. http://www.ers.usda.gov/Briefing/FoodSecurity/measurement.htm. Retrieved on 2008-02-23.

12. Melaku Ayalew–<u>What is Food Security and Famine and Hunger?</u>

13 Community Food Security Coalition, What is community food security? http://www.foodsecurity.org/views_cfs_faq.html accessed on November 1, 2007 @ 7:10pm PDT.

14. <u>America's Second Harvest - Hunger and Poverty Statistics</u>

15. Food –immunity-boosting - Source: Daniel Reid, The Tao of Health, Sex and Longevity.

WEBSITES REFERENCES

Environmental Health Perspectives - http://www.ehponline.org/

Hazardous Substances - http://www.chemicalinjury.net/hazardoussubstances.htm